OSTEOPOROSIS DIET COOKBOOK FOR SENIORS

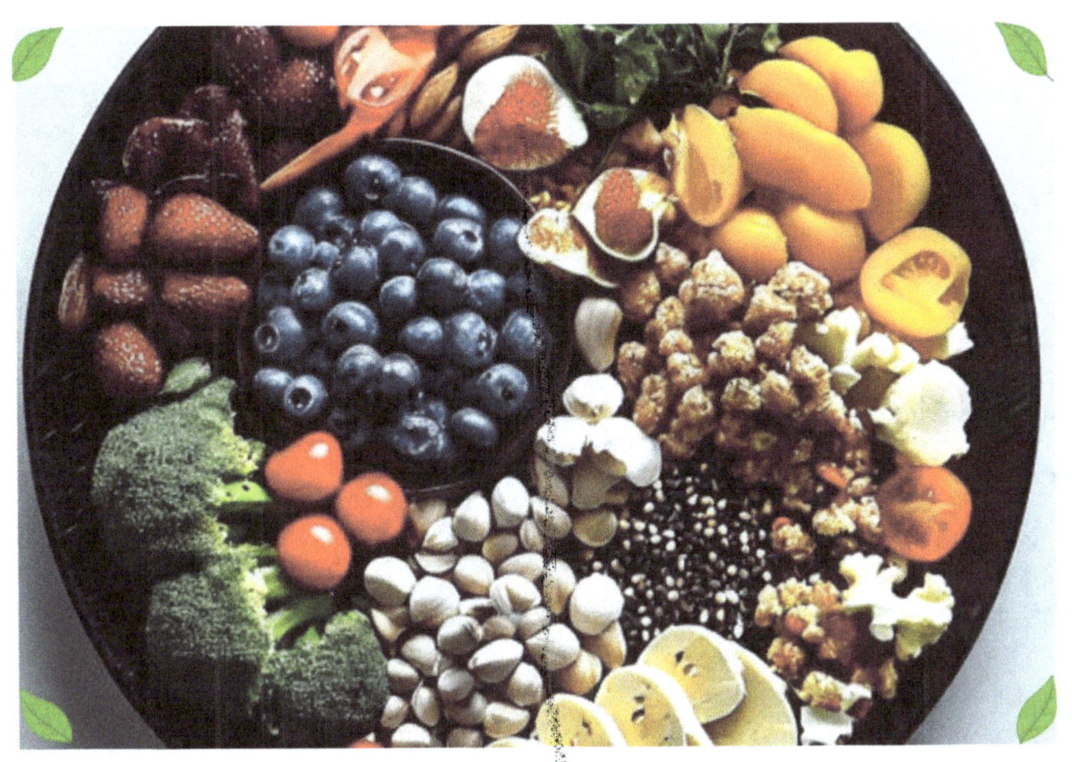

Discover Easy and Delicious Recipes to Prevent and Reverse Bone Loss Naturally and Promoting Bone Health for Older Men and Women

Dr. Kathey A. Moore

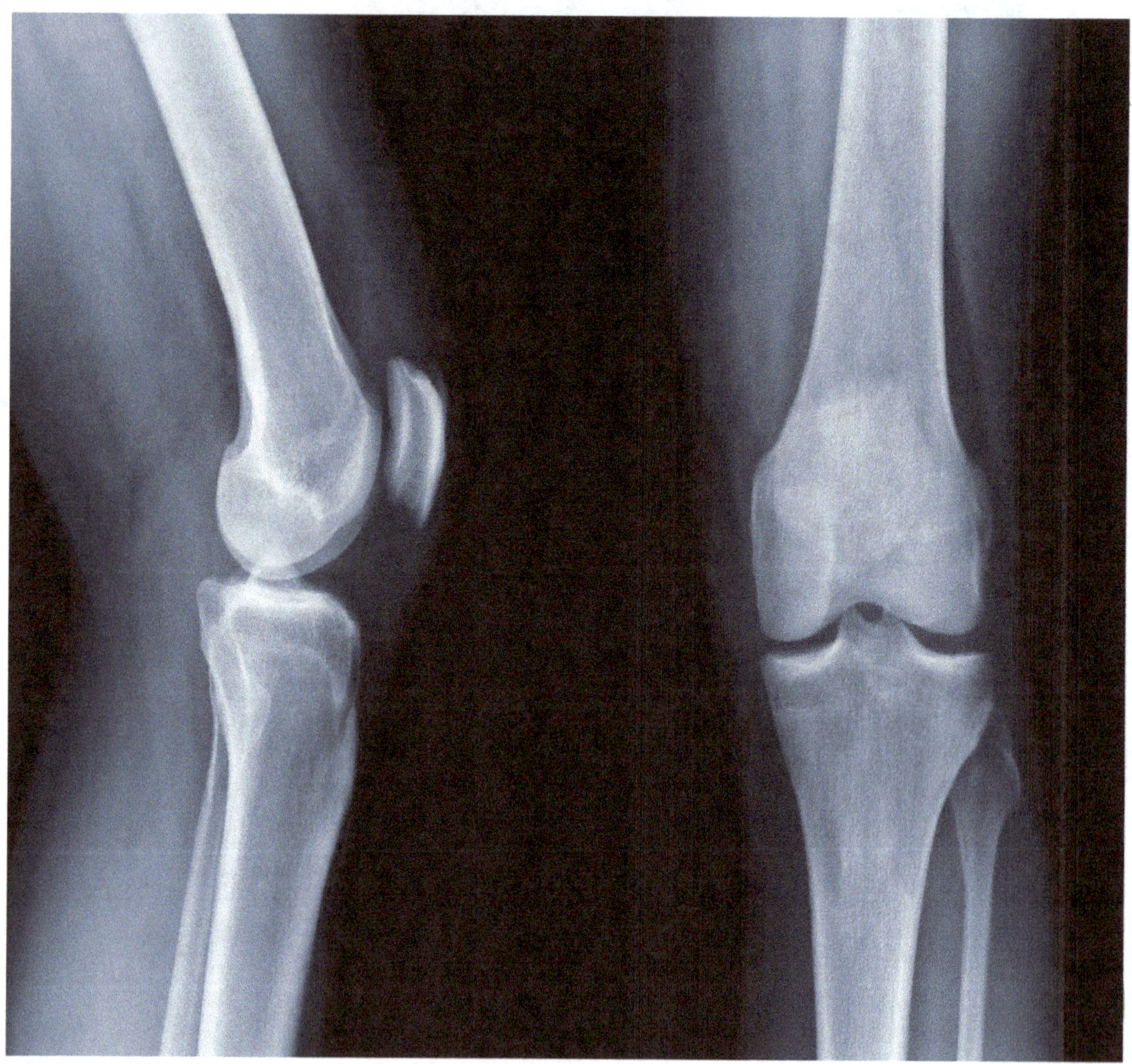

TABLE OF CONTENTS

DEDICATION...4

INTRODUCTION...5

CHAPTER 1 6

    Understanding Osteoporosis 6

    What is Osteoporosis in simple Term? 6

    Types of Osteoporosis 6

    Symptoms of Osteoporosis 7

    Causes and Risk Factors of Osteoporosis 7

    Prevention of Osteoporosis..9

    Importance of Nutrition in Managing Osteoporosis............9

CHAPTER 1: THE ESSENCE OF AN OSTEOPOROSIS DIET COOKBOOK FOR SENIORS 11

    What to Eat, Limit and Avoid 12

    Complications of Osteoporosis if the Right Diet is not followed 13

CHAPTER 2: STRENGTHENING AND HEALING BREAKFAST RECIPES 15

CHAPTER 3: ESSENTIAL LUNCH RECIPES 27

CHAPTER 4: DINNER RECIPES... 43

CHAPTER 5: SNACKS FOR BONE HEALTH RECIPES 60

CHAPTER 6: JUICE AND SMOOTHIE RECIPES 67

CHAPTER 7: DESSERTS FOR BONE HEALTH RECIPES 75

7 DAYS MEAL PLAN... 85

CONCLUSION 90

DEDICATION

For all individuals battling with Osteoporosis,

This book is dedicated to you, the courageous people who face the challenges of osteoporosis with resilience and determination. Your courage in confronting this condition inspires us all. May the recipes and insights in these pages serve as a source of hope and empowerment on your journey towards stronger bones and improved well-being? Your tenacity exemplifies the human spirit, and I dedicate this book to you with much affection and support. Here's to nourishing your body, raising your spirits, and prospering in the face of challenges.

With warmth and gratitude,

Dr. Kathey A. Moore

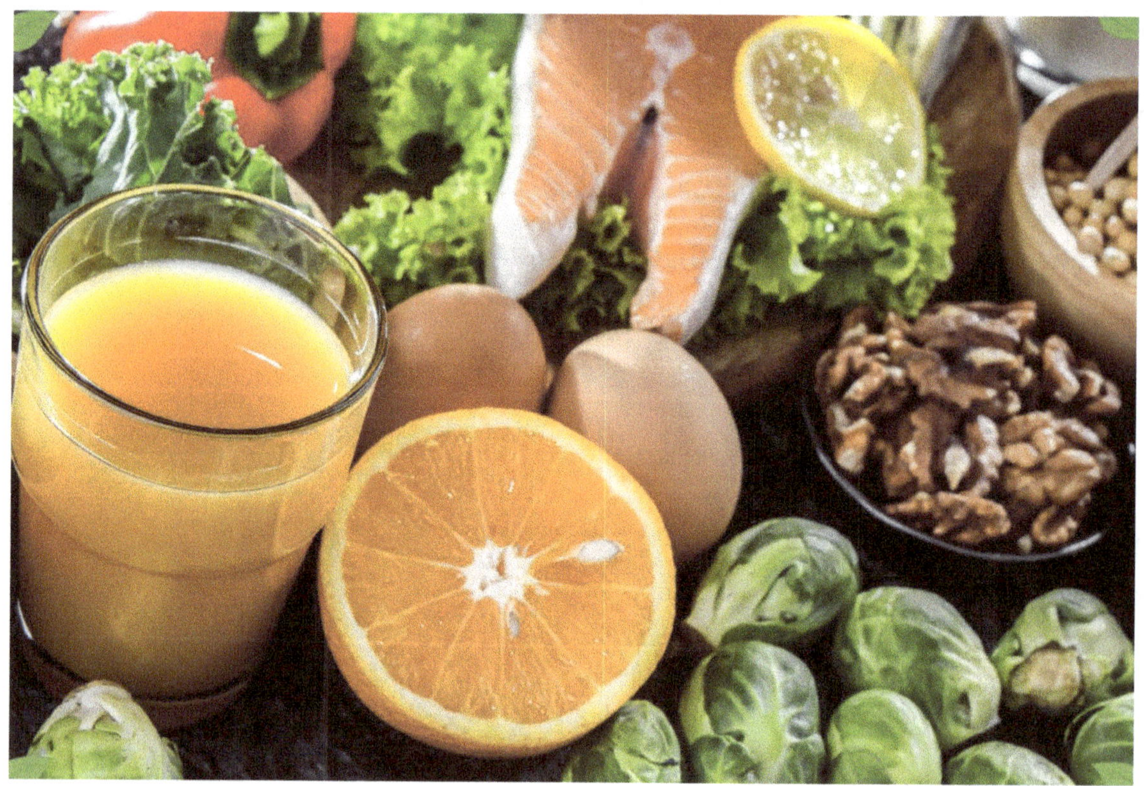

INTRODUCTION

Greetings,

I am Dr. Kathey A. Moore, it is with great pleasure that I welcome you to the "Osteoporosis Diet Cookbook for Seniors." As a dedicated nutrition practitioner, I've had the opportunity to walk alongside countless people dealing with the problems of osteoporosis. Through my experiences, I have witnessed both the hardships and accomplishments that come with this illness, instilling in me a strong desire to provide support and assistance to others in need.

Allow me to tell you the story of Elizabeth, a determined senior who faced the challenges of osteoporosis later in life. Plagued by fractures and the looming threat of bone fragility, Elizabeth sought relief by learning how to take control of her health and strengthen her body's resilience. Elizabeth started on an empowering journey, rediscovering her vigor and enthusiasm for life, thanks to specific nutritional interventions and a newfound respect for the healing power of food.

I express my heartfelt sympathies to everyone dealing with the complications of osteoporosis. Fear of fractures, uncertainty about the future, and interruptions in daily life can all hurt one's spirit. However, behind these limitations comes an opportunity: the ability to harness the transforming power of nutrition to nourish our bodies from the inside.

This cookbook is a light of hope amidst the turbulent waters of osteoporosis. Within its pages, you will find an abundance of healthy recipes that have been carefully crafted to refill your body with the vital nutrients required for good bone health. From calcium-rich treats to protein-packed indulgences and antioxidant-infused wonders, each meal exemplifies nutrition's significant impact on resilience and vitality.

Remember that you are not alone on this gastronomic journey. Armed with information, fed with healthful foods, and guided by the wisdom found within these pages, you can rewrite your health story. Let this cookbook be your constant companion, providing you with the tools and motivation you need to face the challenges of osteoporosis with elegance and resolve.

Let us embrace nutrition's transforming power to create a future full of strength, resilience, and vibrant well-being. Here's to your health, dear reader; may each recipe in these pages be a stepping stone to a life lived to its full potential.

CHAPTER 1

Understanding Osteoporosis

Osteoporosis is a degenerative bone disease characterized by decreased bone density and quality, which increases the risk of fractures. This disorder frequently stays unnoticed until a fracture, usually in the hip, spine, or wrist.

Understanding osteoporosis begins with identifying its underlying causes and risk factors. Aging is a major factor because bone density normally declines with age, particularly in postmenopausal women due to hormonal changes. Furthermore, a lack of calcium and vitamin D in the diet, sedentary lifestyle, smoking, excessive alcohol intake, and certain medical conditions or drugs can all contribute to bone loss.

The implications of osteoporosis go beyond physical discomfort, affecting a person's mobility, independence, and general quality of life. Osteoporosis-related fractures can cause persistent discomfort, disability, and even death, especially in older persons. Thus, early detection and proactive management are critical in minimizing the impact of this condition. Individuals can optimize bone health and lower their risk of fractures by making lifestyle changes such as eating a balanced diet rich in calcium and vitamin D, exercising regularly, quitting smoking, and reducing alcohol use.

What is Osteoporosis in Simple Term?

Osteoporosis is a disorder in which bones become weak and brittle, increasing their likelihood of breaking or fracturing.

Types of Osteoporosis

There are two main forms of osteoporosis:

Primary Osteoporosis: The most prevalent kind is primary osteoporosis, which arises naturally as people age. It primarily affects menopausal and postmenopausal women, as well as older men.

In women, the drop in estrogen levels following menopause increases bone loss, increasing the risk of osteoporosis.

Men's testosterone levels gradually fall with age, contributing to bone loss and increasing the risk of osteoporosis.

Primary osteoporosis can also occur in those who have a family history of osteoporosis, a low body weight, a sedentary lifestyle, or insufficient calcium and vitamin D intake.

Secondary Osteoporosis: Secondary osteoporosis develops as a result of underlying medical disorders or drugs that impair bone health.

Secondary osteoporosis can be caused by hormonal disorders (such as hyperthyroidism or Cushing's syndrome), gastrointestinal disorders (such as celiac disease or inflammatory bowel disease), rheumatic disorders (such as rheumatoid arthritis), and chronic kidney or liver disease.

Corticosteroids (used to treat asthma or autoimmune illnesses), long-term use of proton pump inhibitors (PPIs), and certain anticonvulsant drugs can all lead to secondary osteoporosis by interfering with bone metabolism and calcium absorption.

Understanding the kind of osteoporosis is critical for accurate diagnosis and therapy, as treatment options differ based on the underlying cause.

Symptoms of Osteoporosis

Osteoporosis symptoms are often not obvious until a fracture occurs. However, some people may notice modest indicators of bone loss or weakness. Common signs of osteoporosis include:

Back Pain: Osteoporosis-related fractures in the spine (vertebrae) can result in persistent, dull, or severe back pain. This pain may become worse with movement, bending, or lifting.

Loss of Height: Compression fractures in the spine can cause a gradual loss of height over time. Individuals with osteoporosis may experience a reduction in stature or a stooped posture (kyphosis).

Fractures: Osteoporosis raises the risk of fractures, especially in the hip, spine, and wrist. Fractures can occur with minor trauma or from everyday activity including lifting, bending, or coughing.

Reduced Mobility: Fractures and bone weakening caused by osteoporosis can restrict movement and limit physical activities. People may have trouble walking, climbing stairs, or performing ordinary duties.

Bone Deformities: Severe osteoporosis can cause bone malformations, especially in the spine. These abnormalities can cause a hunched or rounded upper back (kyphosis), as well as a forward head position.

It's crucial to understand that osteoporosis can progress silently, with no visible signs until a fracture occurs. Individuals at risk of osteoporosis, such as postmenopausal women, older adults, and those with risk factors, should have regular screenings and bone density testing to detect bone loss early and avoid fractures. Prompt diagnosis and suitable management can help osteoporosis patients avoid problems and enhance their quality of life.

Causes and Risk Factors of Osteoporosis

Osteoporosis is a complex disorder caused by genetic, hormonal, behavioral, and environmental factors.

Understanding the causes and risk factors linked with osteoporosis is critical for effective prevention and treatment. Here are the main contributors:

Aging: Age is one of the leading causes of osteoporosis. Bone density naturally diminishes with age, making bones more fracture-prone.

Gender: Women have a larger risk of getting osteoporosis than males, especially after menopause. The drop in estrogen levels following menopause hastens bone loss, contributing to the development of osteoporosis.

Hormonal Changes: Imbalanced hormones can have an impact on bone health. Reduced amounts of estrogen in women and testosterone in men can cause bone loss. Hyperthyroidism and Cushing's disease, which alter hormone levels, can both raise the risk of osteoporosis.

Family History: Individuals with a family history of osteoporosis or fractures are more likely to develop the disorder. Genetic factors influence bone density and fracture susceptibility.

Low body weight, sometimes known as underweight, is connected with lower bone density and an increased risk of osteoporosis. Individuals with a low BMI may have insufficient bone mass to support their skeletal structure.

Poor Nutrition: Inadequate calcium and vitamin D intake, both of which are critical minerals for bone health, can lead to osteoporosis. Diets deficient in calcium-rich foods and vitamin D-fortified goods may decrease bone development and retention.

Sedentary Lifestyle: A lack of weight-bearing exercise and physical activity can weaken bones and speed up bone loss. Regular exercise promotes bone production, which helps to maintain bone density and strength.

Smoking and Excessive Alcohol Intake: This can disrupt bone remodeling processes, resulting in lower bone density and an increased risk of fracture.

Long-term usage of drugs including corticosteroids, anticonvulsants, and some cancer treatments can damage bones and contribute to osteoporosis. Medical diseases such as rheumatoid arthritis, inflammatory bowel disease, and chronic kidney or liver illness can all affect bone health.

Individuals who address these risk factors through lifestyle changes, adequate nutrition, exercise, and medical management can lower their risk of developing osteoporosis and maintain excellent bone health for the rest of their lives. Regular screening and bone density testing are critical for early identification and treatment.

Prevention of Osteoporosis

Preventing osteoporosis entails taking a proactive approach to maintaining bone health and lowering the risk of fracture. Here are some important measures for preventing osteoporosis.

Calcium-Rich Diet: Getting enough calcium is critical for developing and maintaining strong bones. Consume calcium-rich foods such as dairy products (milk, yogurt, and cheese), leafy green vegetables (kale, broccoli), fortified cereals, and nuts in your diet.

Vitamin D: Vitamin D is necessary for calcium absorption and bone health. Spending time outside in the sun, eating vitamin D-enriched meals (e.g., fatty fish, fortified dairy products), or taking vitamin D supplements as needed will all help you get enough of the vitamin.

Regular Exercise: Regular Exercise is recommended to increase bone density and strength. Walking, running, dancing, weightlifting, and strength training all promote bone growth and lower the risk of fractures.

Maintain a Healthy Weight: A healthy body weight is achieved by balanced nutrition and regular physical activity. Being underweight or overweight increases the risk of osteoporosis, therefore aim for a healthy BMI.

Limit your alcohol consumption and avoid smoking, as both can weaken bones and raise the chance of fractures. Quitting smoking and limiting alcohol consumption can help keep bones healthy.

Prevent Falls: Take precautions to avoid falls and lower your chance of fracture. Keep your home well-lit and clear of tripping hazards, build handrails and grab bars in restrooms and stairwells, wear supportive footwear, and use assistive equipment as needed.

Regular Bone Density Testing: Talk to your doctor about your risk factors for osteoporosis, and consider getting bone density testing (a DEXA scan) to check your bone health. Early identification of bone loss enables timely intervention and therapy.

Medication Management: If you have underlying medical conditions or use medications that enhance your risk of osteoporosis, consult with your doctor to monitor and manage these variables. They may offer medications or treatments to assist preserve bone density and lower the risk of fractures.

Individuals who follow these preventive steps can lower their risk of getting osteoporosis and retain strong, healthy bones as they age. It is never too early or too late to focus on bone health and implement proactive preventative measures.

Importance of Nutrition in Managing Osteoporosis

Nutrition is critical in controlling osteoporosis because it has a direct impact on bone health and can help slow disease development. Here's why nutrition is important in the treatment of osteoporosis:

Calcium and Vitamin D: Calcium is the fundamental structural component of bones, and enough intakes is required to maintain bone density and strength. Vitamin D is essential for calcium absorption and use in the body. A diet high in calcium and vitamin D promotes bone health and lowers the incidence of fractures.

Bone development and remodeling require nutrients such as protein, magnesium, phosphorus, and vitamin K. Protein forms the structural basis for bones, whereas magnesium and phosphorus aid in bone formation. Vitamin K regulates calcium deposition in bones, which improves bone density and lowers the incidence of fractures.

Bone Loss Prevention: Potassium, vitamin C, and antioxidants all help to protect bone mass and prevent bone loss caused by age and osteoporosis. Potassium-rich meals neutralize acids that can leach calcium from bones, but vitamin C stimulates collagen formation, which supports bone structure.

Muscle Health: Strong muscles contribute to bone health by providing stability and lowering the incidence of falls and fractures. Adequate protein consumption is essential for muscle maintenance and regeneration, preventing muscular weakening and frailty caused by osteoporosis.

Inflammation and Bone Health: Chronic inflammation can cause bone loss and osteoporosis. Anti-inflammatory foods including omega-3 fatty acids, antioxidants (such vitamins C and E), and polyphenols all serve to reduce inflammation and promote bone health.

Overall Health and Well-being: A nutrient-dense, balanced diet promotes overall health and well-being, which is critical for osteoporosis management. Nutrient-dense foods provide critical vitamins, minerals, and antioxidants that promote immunological function, cardiovascular health, and overall well-being.

Medication Effectiveness: Proper nutrition can improve the effectiveness of osteoporosis drugs. Calcium and vitamin D supplements, for example, may increase the effectiveness of osteoporosis drugs like bisphosphonates.

Individuals can promote bone health, slow the progression of osteoporosis, and lower their risk of fractures by eating a nutrient-dense diet rich in calcium, vitamin D, protein, magnesium, phosphorus, vitamin K, potassium, antioxidants, and anti-inflammatory minerals. Nutrition, when combined with regular exercise, medication control, and lifestyle changes, is critical for comprehensive osteoporosis care.

CHAPTER 1: THE ESSENCE OF AN OSTEOPOROSIS DIET COOKBOOK FOR SENIORS

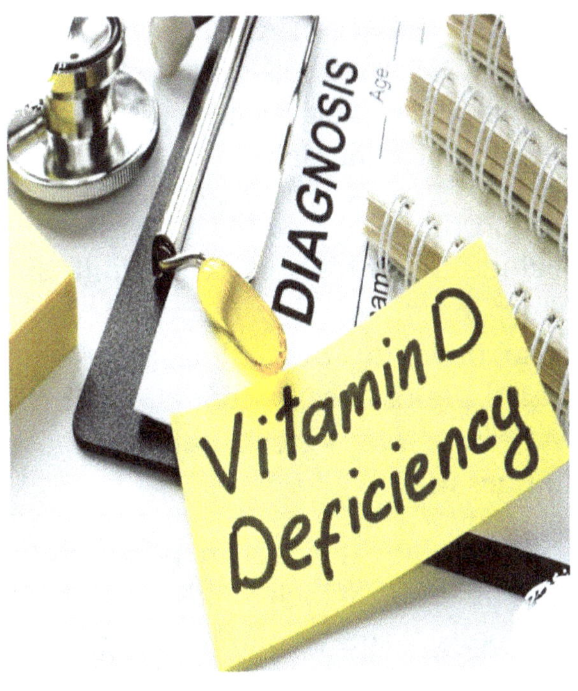

The cornerstone of an osteoporosis diet cookbook for seniors is its capacity to provide people with the knowledge and skills they need to enhance their bone health through delicious and nutritious meals. This specialized cookbook is an invaluable resource for seniors navigating the intricacies of osteoporosis, providing a carefully curated collection of dishes meant to build bone strength, minimize fracture risk, and improve overall well-being.

At its foundation, an osteoporosis diet cookbook acknowledges seniors' special nutritional demands and the need for a well-balanced diet to control the condition. By emphasizing nutrient-rich components such as calcium, vitamin D, protein, magnesium, and antioxidants, the cookbook provides readers with the necessary building blocks for strong and healthy bones. Each recipe is deliberately designed to provide these essential nutrients, allowing seniors to enjoy gourmet meals while prioritizing bone health.

Furthermore, an osteoporosis diet cookbook goes beyond only nutrition, emphasizing the fun and pleasure of eating. With a variety of enticing meals ranging from nourishing soups and salads to fulfilling main courses and scrumptious desserts, the cookbook invites seniors to enjoy the culinary experience and embrace a wide range of flavors and textures. By making healthy eating pleasurable and accessible, the cookbook encourages a positive relationship with food and long-term commitment to a bone-friendly diet.

Additionally, an osteoporosis diet cookbook is a useful tool for meal planning and preparation, providing helpful recommendations, guidelines, and meal ideas customized to the unique needs of seniors with osteoporosis. Whether it's incorporating calcium-rich foods into breakfast smoothies, making protein-packed lunches, or enjoying antioxidant-rich desserts as a treat, the cookbook gives seniors the tools they need to make informed dietary choices and cultivate habits that promote bone health.

Finally, the core of an osteoporosis diet cookbook for seniors is its ability to motivate and empower people to take control of their health and well-being through the transformational power of nutrition. Seniors can improve their quality of life, minimize their risk of fractures, and embark on a journey to stronger, healthier bones for years to come by adopting a diet rich in bone-supporting elements and eating delicious, nourishing meals.

What to Eat, Limit and Avoid

When suffering from osteoporosis, it is critical to make dietary choices that promote bone health while reducing variables that lead to bone loss or fracture risk. Here's a guide for what to eat, restrict, and avoid:

What to Eat?

Calcium-Rich Foods: Include calcium-rich foods in your diet to improve bone strength. Dairy products (milk, yogurt, cheese), leafy green vegetables (kale, collard greens, broccoli), tofu, almonds, and canned fish with bones (such as salmon and sardines) are other examples.

Vitamin D Sources: Make sure you get enough vitamin D to help your body absorb calcium and keep your bones healthy. Consume fatty fish (salmon, mackerel, tuna), egg yolks, fortified dairy products, fortified cereals, and mushrooms.

Protein: Consume enough protein to preserve muscular health and bone density. Choose lean protein sources including chicken, fish, beans, lentils, tofu, and low-fat dairy products.

Magnesium and Phosphorus: Include foods high in magnesium and phosphorus, which are required for bone mineralization. Nuts and seeds, whole grains, beans, lentils, shellfish, and dark leafy greens are all good sources.

Vitamin K: Include meals high in vitamin K, which aids in bone metabolism and calcium management. Choose leafy green vegetables (kale, spinach, collard greens), broccoli, Brussels sprouts, and fermented foods such as sauerkraut.

Antioxidant-Rich Foods: Eating antioxidant-rich foods can help reduce inflammation and protect bone health. Include fruits (berries, citrus fruits), vegetables (tomatoes, bell peppers), almonds, seeds, and olive oil in your meals.

What to Limit:

Sodium: Limit your intake of high-sodium foods, as much sodium can cause calcium loss from bones. Reduce your intake of processed and packaged foods, canned soups, salty snacks, and fast food.

Caffeine: Limit your intake of caffeinated beverages, as much caffeine can interfere with calcium absorption and contribute to bone loss. Limit your coffee, tea, and caffeinated beverage intake.

Limit alcohol consumption because it might weaken bones and raise the risk of fractures. Aim for moderation and restrict alcohol consumption to one drink per day for women and two for men.

What to Avoid:

Sugary Foods and Beverages: These should be consumed in moderation since they contain empty calories and may displace nutrient-rich foods in the diet. Reduce your consumption of sugary snacks, sweets, and sweetened beverages.

High-Phosphorus Foods: Limit your intake of phosphorus-rich foods, especially phosphorus additives found in processed foods and carbonated beverages. Excess phosphorus can impair calcium absorption and compromise bone health.

Smoking: Avoid smoking and secondhand smoke because it has been shown to accelerate bone loss and increase the risk of fracture. Seek help and resources to quit smoking, if necessary.

Individuals with osteoporosis can improve their overall health by adhering to these dietary guidelines and making informed decisions about what to eat, restrict, and avoid. Consult a healthcare physician or certified dietitian for specialized nutrition recommendations based on your specific needs and health objectives.

Complications of Osteoporosis if the Right Diet is not followed

Failure to follow the proper diet for managing osteoporosis can result in a variety of consequences that worsen the condition's progression and raise the risk of fractures. Here are the probable problems of osteoporosis if the proper diet is not followed.

Increased Fracture Risk: Osteoporosis weakens bones, making them more likely to fracture. Without an appropriate intake of key minerals such as calcium, vitamin D, protein, and other bone-supporting elements, bone density may drop further, increasing the risk of fractures from minor trauma or falls.

Progressive Bone Loss: Without sufficient nourishment, bone remodeling processes may be disrupted, resulting in rapid bone loss. Inadequate calcium, vitamin D, magnesium, and other bone-healthy minerals can cause bone loss and weakening over time.

Poor nutrition can cause muscle weakness and imbalance, increasing the risk of falls and fractures. Adequate protein consumption is required to maintain muscle mass and strength, which is critical for bone health and preventing falls.

Fractures in people with osteoporosis may heal more slowly, especially if nutritional inadequacies affect the body's ability to repair and regenerate bone structure. A Proper diet, which includes enough protein, vitamins, and minerals, is critical for good bone healing and regeneration.

Reduced Quality of Life: Complications of untreated or poorly managed osteoporosis, such as fractures, persistent pain, and mobility restrictions, can have a substantial impact on quality of life. Inadequate nutrition exacerbates these issues, causing more physical discomfort, functional impairment, and decreased independence.

Complications from untreated osteoporosis, such as fractures and hospitalizations, can result in significant healthcare costs. Poor nutrition adds to these expenses by delaying recovery, increasing the need for medical interventions, and worsening overall health outcomes.

Secondary Health Issues: Osteoporosis-related fractures and sequelae, especially in older persons, can result in pneumonia, deep vein thrombosis, and pressure ulcers. An Inadequate diet can further weaken the immune system, increasing the likelihood of severe illnesses.

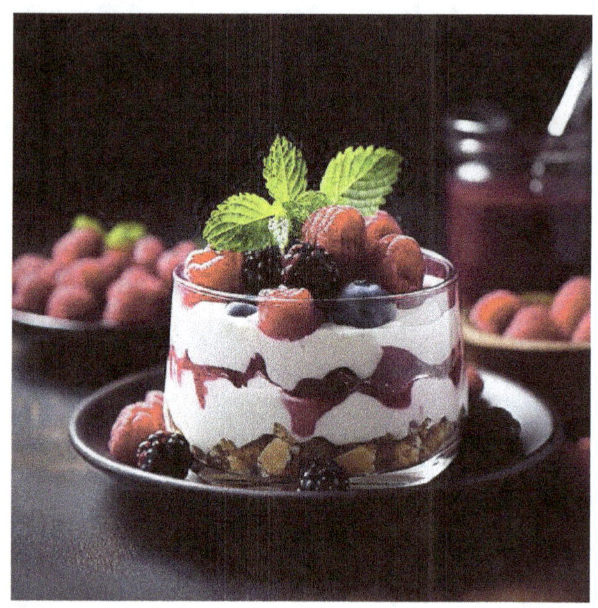

CHAPTER 2: STRENGTHENING AND HEALING BREAKFAST RECIPES

Greek Yogurt and Berry Parfait

Ingredients:

- 1 cup Greek yogurt
- 1/2 cup mixed berries (such as strawberries, blueberries, raspberries)
- 2 tablespoons chopped almonds or walnuts
- 1 tablespoon honey
- 1 teaspoon chia seeds (optional)

Instructions:

- Combine Greek yogurt, berries, and almonds in a glass or bowl.
- Drizzle honey on each layer.
- Optional: add chia seeds on top.

Nutritional Value:

- ✓ Greek yogurt is rich in protein, calcium, and vitamin D.
- ✓ Berries: High in antioxidants and vitamin C.
- ✓ Nuts provide healthful lipids, magnesium, and phosphorus.
- ✓ Honey provides both natural sweetness and antioxidants.
- ✓ Chia seeds provide omega-3 fatty acids and fiber.

Benefit for Osteoporosis: Greek yogurt contains calcium and vitamin D, which are essential for bone health. Berries include antioxidants, which assist to reduce inflammation and improve bone health. Magnesium and phosphorus are found in nuts and help to strengthen and densify bones.

Salmon and Spinach Omelette

Ingredients:

- 2 eggs
- 1/4 cup cooked salmon, flaked
- 1/2 cup fresh spinach leaves
- 1/4 cup diced tomatoes
- 2 tablespoons feta cheese (optional)
- Salt and pepper to taste
- 1 teaspoon olive oil

Instructions:

1. In a mixing bowl, whisk the eggs and season with salt and pepper.
2. In a nonstick skillet, heat the olive oil over medium heat.
3. In the skillet, sauté the spinach and tomatoes until wilted.
4. Pour the beaten eggs over the spinach and tomato.
5. On one half of the omelette, sprinkle with salmon flakes and feta cheese.

6. Once the omelette has set, fold it in half and cook for another minute.
7. Transfer the omelette to a plate and serve hot.

Nutritional Value:

- ✓ Eggs contain protein, vitamin D, and phosphorus.
- ✓ Salmon contains omega-3 fatty acids, vitamin D, and calcium.
- ✓ Spinach provides vitamin K, calcium, and magnesium.
- ✓ Tomatoes provide antioxidants, especially vitamin C.
- ✓ Feta cheese provides calcium and taste.

Benefit for Osteoporosis: This omelette is strong in protein and includes essential nutrients for bone health, including calcium, vitamin D, and vitamin K. Salmon and spinach include omega-3 fatty acids, calcium, and magnesium, all of which promote bone density. Tomatoes and spinach include antioxidants, which assist to reduce inflammation and protect bones.

Calcium-Rich Green Smoothie

Ingredients:

- 1 cup spinach
- 1/2 cup kale
- 1 ripe banana
- 1/2 cup Greek yogurt
- 1 tablespoon almond butter
- 1/2 cup almond milk
- 1 tablespoon chia seeds
- Honey or maple syrup (optional, for sweetness)

Instructions:

1. Blend spinach, kale, banana, Greek yogurt, almond butter, almond milk, and chia seeds in a blender.
2. Blend until it's smooth and creamy.
   If desired, add honey or maple syrup to taste.
3. Pour into a glass and serve instantly.

Nutritional Value:

- ✓ **Spinach and kale:** Excellent sources of calcium, vitamin K, and antioxidants.
- ✓ **Banana:** Provides potassium and natural sweetness.
- ✓ **Greek yogurt:** High in protein and calcium.
- ✓ **Almond butter:** Adds healthy fats, magnesium, and phosphorus.
- ✓ **Chia seeds:** Supply omega-3 fatty acids and additional calcium.

Benefit for Osteoporosis: This green smoothie is high in calcium, vitamin

K, and other nutrients that help bone health.

The combination of leafy greens, Greek yogurt, and chia seeds contains a high calcium concentration, improving bone health and density

Magnesium and phosphorus are important for bone metabolism, and almond butter includes both.

Oatmeal with Almond Milk and Berries

Ingredients:

- 1/2 cup rolled oats
- 1 cup almond milk
- 1/4 cup mixed berries (such as strawberries, blueberries, raspberries)
- 1 tablespoon sliced almonds
- 1 teaspoon honey or maple syrup (optional, for sweetness)
- Pinch of cinnamon (optional)

Instructions:

1. In a small saucepan, combine the rolled oats and almond milk.
2. Cook the oatmeal over medium heat, stirring occasionally, until smooth and creamy.
3. Place the oats in a bowl and top with the berries and chopped almonds.
4. Drizzle with honey or maple syrup and, if desired, sprinkle with cinnamon.
5. Serve heated with relish!

Nutritional value:

- ✓ **Oatmeal:** High in fiber, magnesium, and phosphorus.
- ✓ Almond milk provides calcium and vitamin D.
- ✓ Berries are high in antioxidants and vitamin C.
- ✓ Almonds provide protein, healthy fats, and magnesium.

Benefit for Osteoporosis: This oatmeal recipe is a full and nutritious breakfast option rich in calcium, vitamin D, and antioxidants. Almond milk contains calcium and vitamin D, which are essential for bone health. Berries include antioxidants, which help prevent bone loss and inflammation.

Whole wheat avocado toast with poached egg

Ingredients:

- 2 slices whole wheat bread
- 1 ripe avocado

- 2 eggs
- Salt and pepper to taste
- Red pepper flakes (optional, for spice)
- Fresh parsley or cilantro (optional, for garnish)

Instructions:

1. Toast the whole wheat bread slices till golden brown.
2. Meanwhile, mash the ripe avocado in a bowl and season with salt, pepper, and red pepper flakes to taste.
3. Poach the eggs in boiling water until the whites are hard but the yolks are still runny.
4. Spread the mashed avocado evenly over the toasted bread slices.
5. Carefully place a poached egg on top of each avocado toast.
6. Garnish with fresh parsley or cilantro if desired.

Nutritional Value:

- ✓ Whole wheat bread: Provides fiber, magnesium, and phosphorus.
- ✓ Avocado: Rich in healthy fats, potassium, and vitamin K.
- ✓ Eggs: Good source of protein, vitamin D, and phosphorus.
- ✓ Benefit for Osteoporosis:
- ✓ Avocado toast with poached egg is a nutritious breakfast option that promotes bone health.
- ✓ Whole wheat bread contains fiber and nutrients necessary for bone metabolism.
- ✓ Avocado contains healthful lipids and vitamin K, which aid in bone development and calcium absorption.

Spinach and Mushroom Frittata

Ingredients:

- 6 eggs
- 1 cup fresh spinach leaves
- 1/2 cup sliced mushrooms
- 1/4 cup diced onions
- 1/4 cup grated Parmesan cheese
- Salt and pepper to taste
- 1 tablespoon olive oil

Instructions:

1. Preheat the oven to 350°F (175°C).
   In a mixing bowl, whisk the eggs and season with salt and pepper.
2. Heat the olive oil in an oven-safe skillet over medium heat.
3. Sauté the onions and mushrooms until they soften.
4. Cook the spinach leaves until wilted.
5. Pour the beaten eggs over the vegetables in the skillet.
6. Sprinkle grated Parmesan cheese evenly over the eggs.
7. Bake for 15-20 minutes, or until the frittata is set and golden brown on top.

8. Cut into wedges and serve when hot.

Nutritional Value:

- ✓ Eggs are an excellent source of protein, vitamin D, and phosphorus.
- ✓ Spinach provides vitamin K, calcium, and magnesium.
- ✓ Mushrooms include vitamin D and antioxidants.
- ✓ Parmesan cheese provides calcium and taste.

Benefit for Osteoporosis: This spinach and mushroom frittata is a healthy, calcium-rich meal that promotes bone health. Eggs include protein and vitamin D, which are required to maintain bone density. Spinach and mushrooms include vitamin K and antioxidants, which assist to prevent bone loss.

Blueberry Almond Overnight Oats

Ingredients:

- 1/2 cup rolled oats
- 1/2 cup almond milk
- 1/4 cup Greek yogurt
- 1/4 cup fresh blueberries
- 1 tablespoon almond butter
- 1 tablespoon honey
- 1 tablespoon sliced almonds

Instructions:

1. In a jar or bowl, mix together the rolled oats, almond milk, Greek yogurt, and almond butter.
2. Stir in the fresh blueberries and honey until fully combined.
3. Cover the jar or bowl and refrigerate overnight or at least 4 hours.
4. For added crunch, garnish with sliced almonds before serving.
5. Enjoy chilled or warm in the microwave.

Nutritional value:

- ✓ Rolled oats are high in fiber, magnesium, and phosphorus.
- ✓ Almond milk provides calcium and vitamin D.
- ✓ Greek yogurt is high in protein and calcium.
- ✓ Blueberries provide antioxidants and vitamin C.
- ✓ Almond butter provides healthful lipids, magnesium, and phosphorus.

Benefit for Osteoporosis: Blueberry almond overnight oats are a handy and nutrient-dense breakfast alternative for bone health. Rolled oats include fiber and nutrients necessary for bone metabolism. Almond milk and Greek yogurt include calcium and vitamin D, which are essential for bone density.

Whole Grain Banana Pancakes

Ingredients:

- 1 cup whole wheat flour
- 1 tablespoon baking powder
- 1/4 teaspoon salt
- 1 ripe banana, mashed
- 1 cup almond milk
- 1 egg
- 1 tablespoon honey
- 1 teaspoon vanilla extract
- Use either Cooking spray or butter for greasing the pan

Instructions:

1. In a large mixing basin, combine whole wheat flour, baking powder, and salt.
2. In another bowl, combine the mashed banana, almond milk, egg, honey, and vanilla essence until well blended.
3. Pour the wet ingredients into the dry ingredients and stir until barely combined. Do not over mix; lumps are fine.
4. Place a nonstick skillet or griddle over medium heat and gently grease with cooking spray or butter.
5. Pour about 1/4 cup batter into the skillet per pancake.
6. Cook until bubbles form on the surface, then flip and cook until golden brown on the other side.
7. Serve warm with your preferred toppings, such as sliced bananas, berries, or maple syrup.

Nutritional value:

- ✓ Whole wheat flour contains fiber, magnesium, and phosphorus.
- ✓ Banana provides potassium, fiber, and natural sweetness.
- ✓ Almond milk contains calcium and vitamin D.
- ✓ Honey has natural sweetness and antioxidants.

Benefit for Osteoporosis: These whole-grain banana pancakes are a delightful and nutritious breakfast option that promotes bone health. Whole wheat flour contains fiber and necessary nutrients for bone metabolism. Bananas have potassium, which promotes bone density, while almond milk contains calcium and vitamin D.

Spinach and Mushroom Breakfast Quesadilla

Ingredients:

- 2 whole wheat tortillas
- 1 cup fresh spinach leaves
- 1/2 cup sliced mushrooms
- 1/4 cup shredded cheese (cheddar or mozzarella)
- 2 eggs
- Salt and pepper to taste
- Olive oil for cooking

Instructions:

1. In a medium skillet, heat a tiny amount of olive oil.
2. Sauté the sliced mushrooms until soft.
   Cook the fresh spinach leaves in the skillet until wilted.
3. In a separate skillet, scramble the eggs.
4. Place a tortilla in the skillet and top with half of the shredded cheese.
5. Sprinkle the sautéed mushrooms, spinach, and scrambled eggs on top of the cheese.
6. Sprinkle the remaining cheese over the contents, and then top with the second tortilla.
7. Cook until the bottom tortilla is golden brown, and then carefully turn it to cook the other side.
8. Cut into wedges and serve when hot.

Nutritional Value:

- ✓ Spinach provides calcium, magnesium, and vitamin K.
- ✓ Mushrooms include vitamin D and antioxidants.
- ✓ Eggs contain protein, vitamin D, and phosphorus.
- ✓ Whole wheat tortillas provide fiber and important minerals.

Benefit for Osteoporosis: This breakfast quesadilla offers a balanced combination of protein, calcium, and vitamin D, which are essential for bone health.

Spinach and mushrooms provide nutrients that support bone density and strength.

Whole wheat tortillas contribute fiber, promoting digestive health and overall well-being.

Berry and Spinach Protein Smoothie

Ingredients:

- 1 cup spinach
- 1/2 cup mixed berries (strawberries, blueberries, raspberries)
- 1 scoop protein powder (whey or plant-based)
- 1 tablespoon almond butter
- 1 cup almond milk
- 1 teaspoon honey or maple syrup (optional)

Instructions:

1. Place spinach, mixed berries, protein powder, almond butter, almond milk, and honey or maple syrup (if using) in a blender.
2. Blend until smooth and creamy.
3. Pour into a glass and serve immediately.

Nutritional Value:

- ✓ Spinach: Rich in calcium, magnesium, and vitamin K.
- ✓ Mixed berries are rich in antioxidants and vitamin C.
- ✓ Protein powder: Provides additional protein for muscle and bone health.
- ✓ Almond butter: Source of healthy fats, magnesium, and phosphorus.
- ✓ Almond milk: Supplies calcium and vitamin D.

Benefit for Osteoporosis: This protein smoothie is an easy way to get important nutrients for bone health into your morning. Spinach and berries include antioxidants and vitamins that promote bone density and prevent inflammation. Protein powder and almond butter provide protein and healthy fats, which promote general bone health and muscle strength.

Whole Grain Pancakes with Yogurt and Berries

Ingredients:

- 1 cup whole wheat flour
- 1 tablespoon baking powder
- 1 tablespoon honey or maple syrup
- 1 egg
- 1 cup Greek yogurt
- 1/2 cup mixed berries (strawberries, blueberries, raspberries)
- Olive oil or cooking spray

Instructions:

1. In a mixing bowl, combine whole wheat flour, baking powder, honey or maple syrup, egg, and Greek yogurt.
2. Stir until well combined to form a pancake batter.
3. Place a nonstick skillet over medium heat and lightly coat with olive oil or cooking spray.
4. Pour about 1/4 cup of batter onto the skillet to form pancakes.
5. Cook until bubbles appear on the surface, then flip and cook until golden brown on both sides.
6. Serve the pancakes topped with Greek yogurt and mixed berries.

- ✓ Whole wheat flour contains fiber, magnesium, and phosphorus.
- ✓ Greek yogurt is high in protein and calcium.
- ✓ Mixed berries: High in antioxidants and vitamins C.
- ✓ Honey or maple syrup provides natural sweetness.

Benefit for Osteoporosis: These whole grain pancakes are a delicious and nutritious breakfast option packed with protein, calcium, and antioxidants. Greek yogurt offers calcium and protein, essential for bone health. Berries provide antioxidants that help reduce inflammation and protect bone density.

Quinoa Breakfast Bowl with Almonds and Dried Fruit

Ingredients:

- 1/2 cup cooked quinoa
- 1/4 cup almond milk
- 2 tablespoons sliced almonds
- 2 tablespoons dried apricots, chopped
- 1 tablespoon dried cranberries or raisins
- 1 teaspoon honey or maple syrup (optional)

Instructions:

1. In a bowl, combine cooked quinoa and almond milk.
2. Stir in sliced almonds, chopped dried apricots, and dried cranberries or raisins.
3. If desired, drizzle with honey or maple syrup for added sweetness.
4. Mix well and serve warm or cold.

Nutritional Value:

- ✓ Quinoa is high in protein, calcium, and magnesium.
- ✓ Almond milk provides calcium and vitamin D.
- ✓ Almonds contain healthful lipids, magnesium, and phosphorus.
- ✓ Dried apricots and cranberries provide antioxidants and other minerals.

Benefit for Osteoporosis: This quinoa breakfast bowl contains a nutritious combination of protein, calcium, and antioxidants that promote bone health. Quinoa is a complete protein and an excellent supply of magnesium, which is required for bone metabolism. Almond milk and almonds include calcium and vitamin D, which improve bone health and density.

Chia Seed Breakfast Bowl

Ingredients:

- 2 tablespoons chia seeds
- 1/2 cup almond milk
- 1/2 cup Greek yogurt
- 1/2 cup mixed berries (strawberries, blueberries, raspberries)
- 1 tablespoon honey or maple syrup

Instructions:

1. In a bowl, mix chia seeds and almond milk. Stir well and let sit for 5 minutes.
2. Add Greek yogurt on top of the chia seed mixture.
3. Add mixed berries and drizzle with honey or maple syrup.
4. Stir before eating to combine all ingredients.

Benefit for Osteoporosis: Chia seeds are high in calcium, magnesium, and phosphorus, which are essential for bone health. Greek yogurt provides calcium and protein, supporting bone strength and density. Berries offer antioxidants that help reduce inflammation and protect bone density.

Sweet Potato and Spinach Breakfast Hash

Ingredients:

- 1 medium sweet potato, diced
- 1 cup spinach leaves
- 1/4 cup diced onions
- 2 eggs
- Salt and pepper to taste
- Olive oil for cooking

Instructions:

1. In a medium-size skillet, heat the olive oil.
2. Add diced sweet potato and cook until tender and lightly browned.
3. Add diced onions and spinach leaves to the skillet, and cook until onions are translucent and spinach is wilted.
4. Create two wells in the hash and crack an egg into each well.
5. Cover the skillet and cook until the eggs are cooked to your desired doneness.
6. Season with salt and pepper before serving.

Benefit for Osteoporosis: Sweet potatoes are rich in potassium and vitamin C, which help maintain bone density and collagen production. Spinach provides calcium, magnesium, and vitamin K, supporting bone strength and reducing the risk of fractures. Eggs are a good source of protein, vitamin D, and phosphorus, essential for bone health and maintenance.

Millet Porridge with Almonds and Dates

Ingredients:

- 1/2 cup millet
- 1 1/2 cups water
- 1/4 cup almond milk

- 2 tablespoons sliced almonds
- 2 tablespoons chopped dates
- 1/2 teaspoon cinnamon (optional)

Instructions:

1. Rinse millet under cold water.
2. In a saucepan, bring water to a boil and add millet.
3. Reduce the heat, cover, and simmer for 15-20 minutes, or until the millet is soft.
4. Stir in almond milk, sliced almonds, chopped dates, and cinnamon (if using).
5. Cook for another 2-3 minutes, until well heated.

Benefit for Osteoporosis: Millet is a gluten-free whole grain high in magnesium and phosphorus, which improves bone health and density. Almond milk contains calcium and vitamin D, which are vital elements for bone health. Dates are a natural supply of potassium and magnesium, which promote bone strength and lower the risk of osteoporosis.

Cottage Cheese and Pineapple Breakfast Bowl

Ingredients:

- 1/2 cup cottage cheese
- 1/2 cup diced pineapple
- 2 tablespoons chopped walnuts
- 1 tablespoon honey
- Pinch of cinnamon (optional)

Instructions:

1. In a bowl, combine cottage cheese and diced pineapple.
2. Top with chopped walnuts and drizzle with honey.
3. Sprinkle with cinnamon, if desired.
4. Serve chilled or at room temperature.

Benefit for Osteoporosis: Cottage cheese is high in protein and calcium, supporting bone strength and density. Pineapple provides vitamin C and manganese, which aid in collagen synthesis and bone formation. Walnuts offer omega-3 fatty acids and antioxidants, reducing inflammation and supporting overall bone health.

Egg and Spinach Breakfast Wrap

Ingredients:

- 2 large eggs
- 1 cup fresh spinach leaves
- 2 whole wheat tortillas
- 1/4 cup shredded cheese (cheddar or mozzarella)
- Salt and pepper to taste
- Olive oil for cooking

Instructions:

1. Warm olive oil in a skillet over medium heat.
2. Add fresh spinach leaves and sauté until wilted.
3. Push the spinach to one side of the skillet and crack the eggs into the other side.

4. Scramble the eggs until cooked through, and then mix with the spinach.
5. Warm the whole wheat tortillas in the skillet.
6. Divide the egg and spinach mixture between the tortillas.
7. Sprinkle shredded cheese over the filling.
8. Roll up the tortillas and serve hot.

Benefit for Osteoporosis: Eggs are rich in protein and vitamin D, essential for bone health and calcium absorption. Spinach provides calcium, vitamin K, and magnesium, supporting bone density and reducing the risk of fractures. Whole wheat tortillas offer fiber and nutrients that promote digestive health and overall well-being.

Avocado and Tomato Breakfast Toast

Ingredients:

- 2 slices whole grain bread, toasted
- 1 ripe avocado, mashed
- 1 medium tomato, sliced
- 1 tablespoon chopped fresh basil
- Salt and pepper to taste
- Optional: a drizzle of balsamic glaze

Instructions:

1. Spread mashed avocado evenly on each slice of toasted bread.
2. Arrange tomato slices on top of the avocado.
3. Sprinkle chopped fresh basil over the tomatoes.
4. Season with salt and pepper to taste.
5. Drizzle with balsamic glaze if desired.
6. Serve immediately.

Benefit for Osteoporosis: Avocado is rich in vitamin K, which aids in calcium absorption and bone mineralization. Tomatoes provide vitamin C and lycopene; antioxidants that help reduce bone loss and maintain bone density. Whole grain bread offers fiber and nutrients that support digestive health and overall well-being.

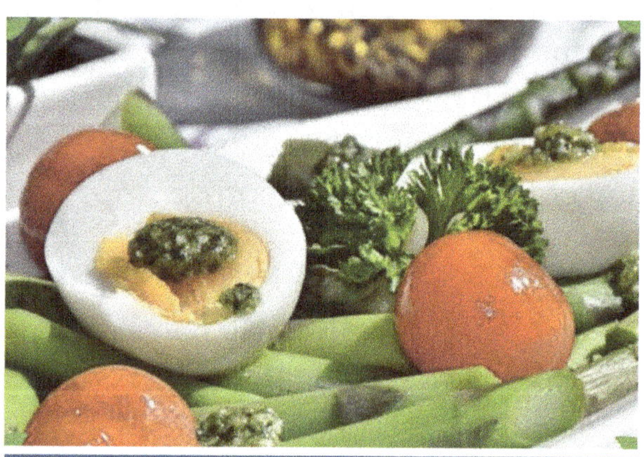

CHAPTER 3: ESSENTIAL LUNCH RECIPES

Salmon and Quinoa Salad

Ingredients:

- 1 cup cooked quinoa
- 4 oz grilled salmon fillet
- 2 cups mixed greens (spinach, kale, arugula)
- 1/2 cup cherry tomatoes, halved
- 1/4 cup sliced cucumber
- 1/4 cup sliced almonds
- 2 tablespoons feta cheese (optional)
- 1 tablespoon olive oil
- 1 tablespoon lemon juice
- Salt and pepper to taste

Instructions:

1. In a large mixing bowl, add the cooked quinoa, mixed greens, cherry tomatoes, cucumber, sliced almonds, and feta cheese (if using).
2. Toss the salad with olive oil and lemon juice.
3. Season with salt and pepper to taste.
4. Place a grilled salmon fillet on top of the salad.

Nutritional Value:

- ✓ Salmon contains omega-3 fatty acids, vitamin D, and calcium.
- ✓ Quinoa is high in protein, magnesium, and phosphorus.
- ✓ Mixed greens provide vitamin K, calcium, and antioxidants.
- ✓ Cherry tomatoes and cucumbers provide vitamins and minerals.
- ✓ Almonds contain healthful lipids, magnesium, and phosphorus.
- ✓ Olive oil contains monounsaturated fats and antioxidants.
- ✓ Feta cheese provides calcium and taste.

Benefit for Osteoporosis: This salmon and quinoa salad contains vital elements for bone health, such as omega-3 fatty acids, calcium, and vitamin D. Quinoa contains protein and magnesium, which help to maintain bone strength and density. Leafy greens include vitamin K, which is essential for bone metabolism and calcium absorption.

Grilled chicken and vegetable stir fry

Ingredients:

- 6 oz boneless, skinless chicken breast, sliced
- 2 cups mixed vegetables (bell peppers, broccoli, carrots)
- 1/2 cup snow peas
- 2 cloves garlic, minced

- 2 tablespoons soy sauce (low-sodium)
- 1 tablespoon olive oil
- 1 teaspoon sesame oil
- 1 tablespoon sesame seeds
- Cooked brown rice or quinoa (optional, for serving)

Instructions:

1. Heat the olive oil in a large skillet or wok over medium-high heat.
2. Cook the sliced chicken breast and minced garlic in the skillet until they are browned and cooked through.
3. Stir-fry the mixed veggies and snow peas in the skillet until soft and crisp.
4. Drizzle soy sauce and sesame oil over the stir-fry and toss to evenly coat.
5. Cook for a further minute after adding the sesame seeds to the stir fry.
6. Remove from heat and serve hot, with cooked brown rice or quinoa.

Nutritional Value:

- ✓ Chicken breast is an excellent protein, phosphorous, and vitamin B6 source.
- ✓ Mixed veggies offer vitamins, minerals, and antioxidants.
- ✓ Snow peas are high in vitamin C, vitamin K, and fiber.
- ✓ Garlic contains allicin, a chemical with possible bone-protective effects.
- ✓ Soy sauce enhances flavor and provides a small amount of protein.
- ✓ Olive oil and sesame oil provide healthful lipids and flavor.
- ✓ Sesame seeds contain calcium, magnesium, and phosphorus.

Benefit for Osteoporosis: This grilled chicken and vegetable stir-fry is a healthy and tasty dinner that promotes bone health. Chicken breast contains high-quality protein, which is needed for bone density and muscle strength. Vegetables provide a range of vitamins and minerals, including vitamin K, which aids bone metabolism and calcium absorption.

Spinach and Feta Stuffed Bell Peppers

Ingredients:

- 2 bell peppers, halved and seeded
- 2 cups fresh spinach leaves
- 1/2 cup cooked quinoa
- 1/4 cup crumbled feta cheese
- 1/4 cup diced tomatoes
- 1 tablespoon olive oil
- 1 clove garlic, minced
- Salt and pepper to taste

Instructions:

1. Preheat the oven to 375° Fahrenheit (190° Celsius).

2. In a skillet, heat the olive oil over medium heat. Add the minced garlic and cook until fragrant.
3. Cook the spinach in the skillet until it has wilted.
4. Remove the skillet from the heat and mix in the cooked quinoa, chopped tomatoes, and crumbled feta cheese. Season with salt and pepper to taste.
5. Stuff the halved bell peppers with the spinach-quinoa mixture.
6. Place the stuffed bell peppers on a baking tray and bake in a preheated oven for 20-25 minutes, or until soft.
7. Remove from the oven and serve hot.

Nutritional Value:

- ✓ Bell peppers are high in vitamin C, vitamin K, and antioxidants.
- ✓ Spinach provides calcium, magnesium, and vitamin K.
- ✓ Quinoa is high in protein, magnesium, and phosphorus.
- ✓ Feta cheese provides calcium and taste.
- ✓ Tomatoes provide vitamins and antioxidants.
- ✓ Olive oil contains monounsaturated fats and antioxidants.

Benefit for Osteoporosis: This spinach and feta stuffed bell pepper recipe is a nutrient-dense supper that promotes bone health. Spinach and quinoa include calcium, magnesium, and vitamin K, which are necessary for bone density and strength.

Bell peppers are high in vitamin C, which promotes collagen formation, an important component of bone structure.

Lentil and Vegetable Soup

Ingredients:

- 1 cup dried lentils, rinsed and drained
- 4 cups vegetable broth
- 1 onion, diced
- 2 carrots, diced
- 2 celery stalks, diced
- 2 cloves garlic, minced
- 1 teaspoon ground cumin
- 1/2 teaspoon smoked paprika
- Salt and pepper to taste
- Fresh parsley, chopped (for garnish)

Instructions:

1. In a large pot, heat the olive oil over medium heat. Cook the diced onion, carrots, and celery until softened.
2. Cook for another minute, stirring in the minced garlic, ground cumin, and smoky paprika.
3. Add the washed lentils and vegetable broth to the pot. Bring to a boil, then reduce the heat and simmer for 20-25 minutes, or until the lentils are cooked.

4. Season the soup with salt and pepper, to taste.
5. Serve hot and garnish with chopped fresh parsley.

Nutritional Value:

✓ Lentils are an excellent source of protein, fiber, and minerals such as calcium, magnesium, and phosphorous.
✓ Vegetables (onion, carrots, celery) include vitamins, minerals, and antioxidants.
✓ Garlic contains chemicals with possible bone-protective effects.
✓ Spices (cumin, paprika): They enhance flavor and may have anti-inflammatory properties.
✓ Fresh parsley adds freshness while also providing essential vitamins and minerals.

Benefit for Osteoporosis: This lentil and vegetable soup is a nourishing and satisfying meal that promotes bone health. Lentils are a plant-based source of protein and vital minerals that promote bone health and density. Vegetables provide vitamins and antioxidants that help reduce inflammation and promote bone health.

Greek Salad with Grilled Chicken

Ingredients:

• 6 oz grilled chicken breast, sliced
• 2 cups mixed greens (romaine lettuce, cucumber, red onion, olives, cherry tomatoes)
• 1/4 cup crumbled feta cheese
• 2 tablespoons extra virgin olive oil
• 1 tablespoon red wine vinegar
• 1 teaspoon dried oregano
• Salt and pepper to taste
• Lemon wedges (for serving)

Instructions:

1. In a large bowl, combine the mixed greens, cucumber, red onion, olives, and cherry tomatoes.
2. The dressing is made by whisking together extra virgin olive oil, red wine vinegar, dried oregano, salt, and pepper in a small bowl.
3. Drizzle the dressing over the salad and toss to distribute evenly.
4. Top the salad with sliced grilled chicken breast and crumbled feta cheese.
5. Serve lemon slices on the side.

Nutritional Value:

✓ Grilled chicken breast is a good source of protein, phosphorous, and vitamin B6.
✓ Mixed greens and vegetables include vitamins, minerals, and antioxidants.
✓ Feta cheese: Contains calcium and taste.

- ✓ Olive oil contains both monounsaturated fats and antioxidants.
- ✓ Red wine vinegar: Provides acidity and flavor without adding calories.

Benefits for osteoporosis: This Greek salad with grilled chicken is a light and pleasant meal that contains important elements for bone health. Grilled chicken breast contains high-quality protein, which is required to maintain bone density and muscle strength.

Vegetarian Chickpea and Spinach Curry

Ingredients:

- 1 can (15 oz) chickpeas, drained and rinsed
- 2 cups fresh spinach leaves
- 1 onion, finely chopped
- 2 cloves garlic, minced
- 1 tablespoon curry powder
- 1 teaspoon ground turmeric
- 1 can (14 oz) diced tomatoes
- 1 can (13.5 oz) coconut milk
- Salt and pepper to taste
- Cooked brown rice or quinoa (optional, for serving)
- Fresh cilantro, chopped (for garnish)

Instructions:

1. In a large skillet, heat the olive oil over medium heat. Sauté the chopped onion and minced garlic until softened.
2. In the skillet, combine the curry powder and ground turmeric, stirring regularly for approximately a minute until fragrant.
3. Stir in the diced tomatoes and coconut milk, and bring to a simmer.
4. Stir the chickpeas and fresh spinach into the skillet until fully combined.
5. Cook for around 10-15 minutes, until the spinach has wilted and the curry has thickened.
6. Season with salt and pepper to taste.
7. Serve the chickpea and spinach curry hot over cooked brown rice or quinoa, topped with chopped fresh cilantro.

Nutritional Value:

- ✓ Chickpeas: Rich in protein, fiber, calcium, and magnesium.
- ✓ Spinach: Provides calcium, magnesium, and vitamin K.
- ✓ Onion and garlic: Contain sulfur compounds that may support bone health.
- ✓ Tomatoes: Source of vitamin C and antioxidants.
- ✓ Coconut milk: Adds creaminess and healthy fats.

Benefit for Osteoporosis: This vegetarian chickpea and spinach curry has plant-based protein, calcium, and other bone-healthy minerals.

Chickpeas and spinach provide a lot of calcium and magnesium, which are essential for bone density. Turmeric and tomatoes have anti-inflammatory qualities that may help prevent bone loss.

Tuna Salad Stuffed Avocado

Ingredients:

- 2 ripe avocados, halved and pitted
- 1 can (5 oz) tuna, drained
- 1/4 cup diced red bell pepper
- 1/4 cup diced cucumber
- 2 tablespoons chopped fresh parsley
- 2 tablespoons Greek yogurt
- 1 tablespoon lemon juice
- Salt and pepper to taste
- Optional: Sprinkle of paprika or chili flakes for garnish

Instructions:

1. In a mixing bowl, combine the drained tuna, diced red bell pepper, diced cucumber, fresh parsley, Greek yogurt, and lemon juice. Mix well.
2. Season the tuna salad with salt and pepper to taste.
3. Spoon the tuna salad evenly among the halved avocados.
4. Garnish with paprika or chili flakes if preferred.
5. Serve the tuna salad-stuffed avocados.

Nutritional Value:

- ✓ Avocado contains healthful lipids, potassium, and vitamin K.
- ✓ Tuna is rich in protein, omega-3 fatty acids, and vitamin D.
- ✓ Red bell pepper and cucumber include vitamins, minerals, and antioxidants.
- ✓ Greek yogurt: Provides creaminess and extra protein.
- ✓ Lemon juice provides freshness and vitamin C.

Benefit for Osteoporosis: This tuna salad stuffed avocado recipe is a nourishing and filling dinner high in protein, healthy fats, and bone-building elements. Tuna has high levels of vitamin D, which is necessary for calcium absorption and bone health. Avocados include healthful fats and potassium, which may aid in minimizing calcium loss in the urine.

Mediterranean Quinoa Salad

Ingredients:

- 1 cup cooked quinoa
- 1/2 cup chickpeas, drained and rinsed
- 1/2 cup diced cucumber
- 1/2 cup diced tomatoes
- 1/4 cup diced red onion
- 1/4 cup chopped fresh parsley
- 2 tablespoons crumbled feta cheese
- 2 tablespoons extra virgin olive oil
- 1 tablespoon lemon juice

- 1 teaspoon dried oregano
- Salt and pepper to taste

Instructions:

1. In a large mixing bowl, combine cooked quinoa, chickpeas, diced cucumber, tomatoes, red onion, chopped fresh parsley, and feta cheese.
2. Make the dressing by whisking together extra virgin olive oil, lemon juice, dried oregano, salt, and pepper in a small bowl.
3. Pour the dressing over the quinoa salad and toss to coat well.
4. Season with more salt and pepper if necessary.
5. Serve the Mediterranean quinoa salad cold or at room temperature.

Nutritional Value:

- ✓ Quinoa provides protein, fiber, magnesium, and phosphorus.
- ✓ Chickpeas are high in protein, fiber, calcium, and magnesium.
- ✓ Vegetables (cucumber, tomatoes, red onion) provide vitamins, minerals, and antioxidants.
- ✓ Feta cheese provides calcium and taste.
- ✓ Olive oil contains monounsaturated fats and antioxidants.
- ✓ Lemon juice provides freshness and vitamin C.

Benefit for Osteoporosis: This Mediterranean quinoa salad is a nutrient-dense meal that promotes bone health by including protein, calcium, and other critical elements. Quinoa and chickpeas contain plant-based protein and minerals that promote bone health and density. The salad contains antioxidants from veggies and olive oil, which help reduce inflammation and protect bone cells.

Tuna and White Bean Salad

Ingredients:

- 1 can (5 oz) tuna, drained
- 1 can (15 oz) white beans, drained and rinsed
- 1/2 cup diced red bell pepper
- 1/4 cup diced red onion
- 2 tablespoons chopped fresh parsley
- 2 tablespoons olive oil
- 1 tablespoon lemon juice
- Salt and pepper to taste

Instructions:

1. In a large mixing bowl, combine tuna, white beans, diced red bell pepper, diced red onion, and chopped fresh parsley.
2. Drizzle olive oil and lemon juice over the salad.
3. Season with salt and pepper to taste.
4. Toss lightly to combine all ingredients.

Nutritional Value:

- ✓ Tuna is an excellent source of protein, omega-3 fatty acids, and vitamin D.
- ✓ White beans provide protein, fiber, and minerals such as calcium and magnesium.
- ✓ Red bell pepper is high in vitamins C, K, and antioxidants.
- ✓ Red onion contains flavonoids that may help protect bones.
- ✓ Olive oil provides healthful fats and antioxidants.

Benefit for Osteoporosis: Tuna and white bean salad is a protein-packed dish that promotes bone health. Tuna contains vitamin D, which is needed for calcium absorption and bone strength. White beans contain calcium, magnesium, and protein, all of which help to maintain bone density.

Mediterranean Chickpea Salad

Ingredients:

- 1 can (15 oz) chickpeas, drained and rinsed
- 1 cucumber, diced
- 1 cup cherry tomatoes, halved
- 1/4 cup sliced black olives
- 1/4 cup crumbled feta cheese
- 2 tablespoons chopped fresh parsley
- 2 tablespoons extra virgin olive oil
- 1 tablespoon red wine vinegar
- 1 teaspoon dried oregano
- Salt and pepper to taste

Instructions:

In a large mixing bowl, combine chickpeas, diced cucumber, cherry tomatoes, sliced black olives, crumbled feta cheese, and chopped fresh parsley.

The dressing is made by whisking together extra virgin olive oil, red wine vinegar, dried oregano, salt, and pepper in a small bowl.

Pour the dressing over the salad and toss to coat evenly.

Nutritional Value:

- ✓ Chickpeas are an excellent source of protein, fiber, and minerals such as calcium and magnesium.
- ✓ Cucumber and cherry tomatoes offer vitamins, minerals, and hydration.
- ✓ Black olives contain monounsaturated fats and antioxidants.
- ✓ Feta cheese provides calcium and taste.
- ✓ Olive oil contains heart-healthy lipids and antioxidants.

Benefit for Osteoporosis: This Mediterranean chickpea salad is a nutrient-dense meal that improves bone health. Chickpeas are a plant-based source of protein and vital minerals that promote bone strength. Feta cheese and olive oil include calcium and good lipids, which promote bone density and overall wellness.

Vegetable and Lentil Soup

Ingredients:

- 1 cup dried green or brown lentils, rinsed and drained
- 4 cups vegetable broth
- 1 onion, diced
- 2 carrots, diced
- 2 celery stalks, diced
- 2 cloves garlic, minced
- 1 teaspoon ground cumin
- 1/2 teaspoon smoked paprika
- Salt and pepper to taste
- Fresh parsley, chopped (for garnish)

Instructions:

1. In a large pot, heat the olive oil over medium heat. Cook the diced onion, carrots, and celery until softened.
2. Cook for another minute, stirring in the minced garlic, ground cumin, and smoky paprika.
3. Add the washed lentils and vegetable broth to the pot. Bring to a boil, then reduce the heat and simmer for 20-25 minutes, or until the lentils are cooked.
4. Season the soup with salt and pepper, to taste.
5. Serve hot and garnish with chopped fresh parsley.

Nutritional Value:

- Lentils are an excellent source of protein, fiber, and minerals such as calcium, magnesium, and phosphorous.
- Vegetables (onion, carrots, celery) include vitamins, minerals, and antioxidants.
- Garlic contains chemicals with possible bone-protective effects.
- Spices (cumin, paprika): They enhance flavor and may have anti-inflammatory properties.
- Fresh parsley adds freshness while also providing essential vitamins and minerals.

Benefit for Osteoporosis: This vegetable and lentil soup is a nutritious and satisfying meal that promotes bone health. Lentils are a plant-based source of protein and vital minerals that promote bone health and density. Vegetables provide vitamins and antioxidants that help reduce inflammation and promote bone health.

Turkey and Avocado Wrap

Ingredients:

- 4 oz sliced turkey breast
- 1 whole wheat wrap or tortilla
- 1/2 avocado, sliced
- 1/4 cup shredded lettuce
- 2 slices tomato
- 1 tablespoon hummus
- 1 teaspoon Dijon mustard
- Salt and pepper to taste

Instructions:

1. Place the whole wheat wrap or tortilla flat on a clean surface.
2. Spread the hummus and Dijon mustard equally on the wrap.
3. Place sliced turkey breast, avocado slices, shredded lettuce, and tomato slices on top of the wrap.
4. Season with salt and pepper to taste.
5. Roll the wrap tight, folding in the sides as you go.
6. Cut the wrap in half diagonally.
7. Serve immediately or store in foil for later.

Nutritional Value:

- ✓ Turkey breast: Lean source of protein, vitamin B6, and niacin.
- ✓ Avocado: Rich in healthy fats, potassium, and vitamin K.
- ✓ Whole wheat wrap: Provides fiber and essential nutrients.
- ✓ Lettuce and tomato: Add vitamins, minerals, and hydration.
- ✓ Hummus: Contains protein, fiber, and healthy fats.
- ✓ Dijon mustard: Add flavor without extra calories.

Benefit for Osteoporosis: This turkey and avocado wrap is a nutritious and filling lunch that promotes bone health. Turkey breast contains protein and other vital elements that help to maintain bone density and muscle strength.

Avocado contains healthful lipids and vitamin K, which aid in bone metabolism and calcium absorption.

Salmon and Asparagus Quinoa Bowl

Ingredients:

- 4 oz grilled or baked salmon fillet
- 1 cup cooked quinoa
- 1 cup steamed asparagus spears
- 1/4 cup sliced cherry tomatoes
- 2 tablespoons chopped fresh parsley
- 1 tablespoon olive oil
- 1 tablespoon lemon juice
- Salt and pepper to taste

Instructions:

1. In a bowl, combine cooked quinoa, steaming asparagus spears, sliced cherry tomatoes, and chopped fresh parsley.
2. Place the grilled or baked salmon fillet on top of the quinoa bowl.
3. Drizzle olive oil and lemon juice over the bowl.
4. Add salt and pepper to taste.

Nutritional Value:

- ✓ Salmon contains omega-3 fatty acids, vitamin D, and calcium.
- ✓ Quinoa is rich in protein, fiber, and minerals such as magnesium and phosphorus.
- ✓ Asparagus provides vitamin K, folate, and antioxidants.

✓ Cherry tomatoes are high in vitamin C and lycopene.
✓ Olive oil provides healthful fats and antioxidants.

Benefit for Osteoporosis: This salmon and asparagus quinoa bowl is a nutritionally dense meal that promotes bone health.

Salmon contains high levels of vitamin D and omega-3 fatty acids, which are required for calcium absorption and bone strength. Quinoa contains protein and critical minerals that help to preserve bone density.

Vegetable and Tofu Stir-Fry

Ingredients:

- 1 block (14 oz) firm tofu, cubed
- 2 cups mixed vegetables (broccoli, bell peppers, carrots, snap peas)
- 2 cloves garlic, minced
- 2 tablespoons soy sauce (low-sodium)
- 1 tablespoon sesame oil
- 1 tablespoon cornstarch
- 1 tablespoon water
- Cooked brown rice or quinoa (optional, for serving)

Instructions:

1. In a small bowl, combine cornstarch and water to form slurry.
2. Heat the sesame oil in a large skillet or wok over medium-high heat.
3. Add the cubed tofu to the skillet and cook until golden brown on all sides.
4. Stir-fry the minced garlic and mixed vegetables in the skillet until they are soft and crisp.
5. Pour soy sauce over the tofu and vegetables, and then add the cornstarch slurry.
6. Cook for an additional minute, until the sauce thickens.
7. Remove from heat and serve hot, with cooked brown rice or quinoa.

Nutritional value:

✓ Tofu is an excellent source of plant-based protein, calcium, and magnesium.
✓ Mixed veggies offer vitamins, minerals, and antioxidants.
✓ Garlic contains chemicals with possible bone-protective effects.
✓ Soy sauce enhances flavor and provides a little amount of protein.
✓ Sesame oil provides healthful fats and taste.

Benefit for Osteoporosis: This vegetable and tofu stir-fry is a nutrient-dense and pleasant meal that promotes bone health. Tofu is a plant-based calcium and protein source that helps to preserve bone density. Mixed veggies provide a wide range of vitamins and minerals that are essential for bone metabolism and overall health.

Chicken and Vegetable Skewers

Ingredients:

- 6 oz boneless, skinless chicken breast, cut into cubes
- 1 zucchini, sliced
- 1 bell pepper, cut into chunks
- 1 red onion, cut into chunks
- 8 cherry tomatoes
- 2 tablespoons olive oil
- 2 cloves garlic, minced
- 1 tablespoon lemon juice
- 1 teaspoon dried oregano
- Salt and pepper to taste

Instructions:

1. In a mixing dish, add olive oil, garlic, lemon juice, dried oregano, salt, and pepper.
2. Thread chicken chunks and assorted vegetables onto skewers.
3. Brush the skewers with olive oil mixture.
4. Preheat the grill or grill pan to medium-high heat.
5. Grill the skewers for 8-10 minutes, flipping regularly, until the chicken is fully cooked and the veggies are soft.
6. Remove from the grill and serve hot.

Nutritional value:

- ✓ Chicken breast is an excellent source of protein, vitamin B6, and niacin.
- ✓ Zucchini, bell pepper, onion, and cherry tomatoes include vitamins, minerals, and antioxidants.
- ✓ Olive oil provides healthful fats and antioxidants.
- ✓ Garlic and dried oregano enhance flavor and may have anti-inflammatory properties.

Benefits for Osteoporosis: These chicken and vegetable skewers are a delicious and nutritious meal that promotes bone health. Chicken breast contains the high-quality protein required to preserve bone density and muscle strength. Mixed veggies include vitamins and minerals that are essential for bone metabolism and overall well-being.

Salmon and Avocado Salad

Ingredients:

- 4 oz grilled salmon fillet
- 2 cups mixed greens (spinach, arugula, romaine)
- 1/2 avocado, sliced
- 1/4 cup sliced cucumber
- 1/4 cup cherry tomatoes, halved
- 2 tablespoons sliced almonds
- 1 tablespoon extra-virgin olive oil
- 1 tablespoon balsamic vinegar
- Salt and pepper to taste

Instructions:

1. In a large bowl, combine the mixed greens, sliced avocado,

sliced cucumber, cherry tomatoes, and sliced almonds.
2. Top with a cooked salmon fillet.
3. Drizzle extra virgin olive oil and balsamic vinegar over the salad.
4. Season with salt and pepper to taste.

Nutritional value:

- ✓ Salmon contains omega-3 fatty acids, vitamin D, and calcium.
- ✓ Avocado contains healthful lipids, potassium, and vitamin K.
- ✓ Mixed greens provide calcium, magnesium, and vitamin K.
- ✓ Cherry tomatoes and cucumbers are high in vitamins and antioxidants.
- ✓ Almonds contain protein, healthy fats, and calcium.
- ✓ Olive oil with balsamic vinegar: Enhance flavor and provide healthy fats.

Benefit for Osteoporosis: This salmon and avocado salad is high in minerals that promote bone health. Salmon contains omega-3 fatty acids and vitamin D, which improve calcium absorption and bone health. Avocado provides healthful lipids and vitamin K, which are essential for bone metabolism and density.

Quinoa and Vegetable Stir-Fry

Ingredients:

- 1 cup cooked quinoa
- 1 cup mixed vegetables (bell peppers, broccoli, carrots)
- 1/4 cup diced onion
- 2 cloves garlic, minced
- 2 tablespoons low-sodium soy sauce
- 1 tablespoon sesame oil
- 1 tablespoon rice vinegar
- 1 teaspoon grated ginger
- Sesame seeds for garnish

Instructions:

1. Heat the sesame oil in a large skillet over medium heat.
2. Sauté diced onion and minced garlic until aromatic.
3. Stir-fry the mixed vegetables in the skillet until they are soft and crispy.
4. Stir in the cooked quinoa, low-sodium soy sauce, rice vinegar, and grated ginger.
5. Cook for another 2-3 minutes, stirring periodically, until cooked through.
6. Remove from heat and sprinkle with sesame seeds before serving.

Nutritional value:

- ✓ Quinoa is rich in protein, fiber, and minerals such as calcium and magnesium.
- ✓ Mixed veggies offer vitamins, minerals, and antioxidants.
- ✓ Onions and garlic contain chemicals that can protect bones.

✓ Soy sauce enhances flavor and provides a small amount of protein.
✓ Sesame oil provides healthful fats and tastes.
✓ Rice vinegar and ginger provide acidity and depth of flavor.

Benefits for Osteoporosis: This quinoa and vegetable stir-fry is a nutritious and tasty recipe that promotes bone health. Quinoa contains plant-based protein and minerals that are vital for bone strength. Mixed veggies contain vitamins and antioxidants that help reduce inflammation and promote bone health.

Chickpea and Spinach Wrap

Ingredients:

- 1 whole wheat wrap or tortilla
- 1/2 cup cooked chickpeas
- 1/2 cup fresh spinach leaves
- 1/4 cup diced cucumber
- 2 tablespoons diced red bell pepper
- 2 tablespoons hummus
- 1 tablespoon lemon juice
- Salt and pepper to taste

Instructions:

1. Place the whole wheat wrap or tortilla flat on a clean surface.
2. Spread the hummus evenly on the wrap.
3. Place cooked chickpeas, fresh spinach leaves, diced cucumber, and diced red bell pepper on top of the hummus.
4. Drizzle lemon juice over the mixture.
5. Season with salt and pepper to taste.
6. Roll the wrap tight, folding in the sides as you go.
7. Cut the wrap in half diagonally.
8. Serve immediately or store in foil for later.

Nutritional value:

✓ Chickpeas include protein, fiber, and minerals such as calcium and magnesium.
✓ Spinach is high in calcium, magnesium, and vitamin K.
✓ Cucumbers and red bell pepper provide vitamins, minerals, and crunch.
✓ Hummus has protein, healthy fats, and fiber.
✓ Lemon juice: Enhances acidity and freshness.

Benefits for Osteoporosis: This chickpea and spinach wrap is a nutritious and convenient lunch that promotes bone health. Chickpeas include protein and vital minerals that help to maintain bone density. Spinach contains calcium and vitamin K, which are essential for bone metabolism and density.

Mushroom and Spinach Quesadilla

Ingredients:

- 2 whole wheat tortillas
- 1 cup sliced mushrooms
- 2 cups fresh spinach leaves
- 1/2 cup shredded mozzarella cheese
- 1 tablespoon olive oil
- 1/2 teaspoon garlic powder
- Salt and pepper to taste
- Salsa or Greek yogurt (for serving, optional)

Instructions:

1. In a medium-size skillet, heat the olive oil.
2. Cook the sliced mushrooms in the skillet until they soften.
3. Cook the fresh spinach leaves in the skillet until wilted.
4. Season the mushrooms and spinach with garlic powder, salt, and pepper.
5. Remove the skillet from the heat and set aside.
6. Place a whole wheat tortilla on a clean surface.
7. Spread half of the mushroom and spinach mixture evenly on the tortilla.
8. Sprinkle half of the shredded mozzarella cheese over the mushroom and spinach mixture.
9. Place another tortilla on top of the filling.
10. Heat a clean skillet over medium heat and carefully add the quesadilla.
11. Cook for 2-3 minutes per side or until the tortillas are golden brown and the cheese has melted.
12. Remove from the fire and cool for a few minutes before slicing.
13. If desired, serve with a side of salsa or Greek yogurt.

Nutritional value:

- ✓ Mushrooms contain vitamin D and minerals such as selenium and potassium.
- ✓ Spinach is high in calcium, magnesium, and vitamin K.
- ✓ Whole wheat tortillas provide fiber and important minerals.
- ✓ Mozzarella cheese provides calcium and protein.
- ✓ Olive oil contains heart-healthy lipids and antioxidants.

Benefit for Osteoporosis: This mushroom and spinach quesadilla is a tasty and nutritious meal that promotes bone health. Spinach contains calcium and vitamin K, which are essential for bone density and strength. Mushrooms contain vitamin D, which promotes calcium absorption and bone metabolism.

Turkey and Vegetable Stir-Fry

Ingredients:

- 6 oz sliced turkey breast
- 2 cups mixed vegetables (broccoli, bell peppers, carrots)
- 1/4 cup sliced onion
- 2 cloves garlic, minced
- 2 tablespoons low-sodium soy sauce

- 1 tablespoon olive oil
- 1 teaspoon grated ginger
- 1 teaspoon honey
- Sesame seeds for garnish

Instructions:

1. Heat the olive oil in a large skillet or wok over medium heat.
2. Add the sliced onion and minced garlic to the skillet and cook until fragrant.
3. Cook the sliced turkey breast in the skillet until it is browned and well done.
4. Stir-fry the mixed vegetables in the skillet until they are soft and crispy.
5. In a small bowl, combine the low-sodium soy sauce, grated ginger, and honey.
6. Pour the soy sauce mixture onto the turkey and vegetables in the skillet.
7. Cook for another 2-3 minutes, stirring periodically, until cooked through.
8. Remove from heat and sprinkle with sesame seeds before serving.

Nutritional value:

- ✓ Turkey breast is a lean source of protein, vitamin B6, and niacin.
- ✓ Mixed veggies offer vitamins, minerals, and antioxidants.
- ✓ Onions and garlic contain chemicals that can protect bones.
- ✓ Low-sodium soy sauce: Enhances flavor without adding too much sodium.
- ✓ Olive oil provides healthful fats and flavor.
- ✓ Ginger and honey enhance flavor and may have anti-inflammatory properties.

Benefits for Osteoporosis: This turkey and vegetable stir-fry is a balanced and tasty meal that promotes bone health. Turkey breast contains protein and other vital elements that help to maintain bone density and muscle strength. Mixed veggies contain vitamins and antioxidants that help reduce inflammation and promote bone health.

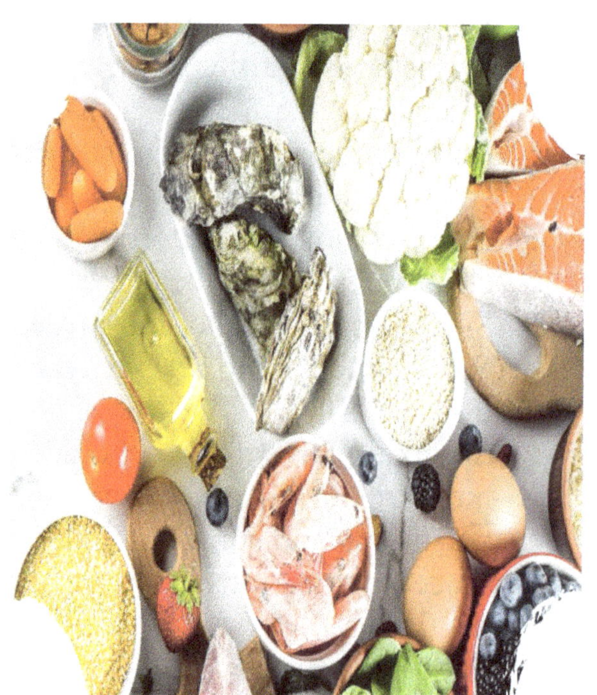

CHAPTER 4: DINNER RECIPES

Grilled Salmon with Roasted Vegetables

Ingredients:

- 4 oz salmon fillet
- 1 cup mixed vegetables (bell peppers, zucchini, carrots)
- 1 tablespoon olive oil
- 1/2 teaspoon dried thyme
- 1/2 teaspoon garlic powder
- Salt and pepper to taste
- Lemon wedges for serving

Instructions:

1. Preheat the grill for medium-high heat.
2. Drizzle olive oil over the salmon fillet, then season with dried thyme, garlic powder, salt, and pepper.
3. In a separate bowl, stir the vegetables with olive oil, salt, and pepper.
4. Place the salmon fillet and mixed veggies on the grill.
5. Grill the salmon for 4-5 minutes on each side, or until cooked through.
6. Grill the mixed veggies for 8–10 minutes, or until tender and slightly browned.
7. Take the salmon and veggies off the grill and serve them hot with lemon wedges on the side.

Nutritional value:

- ✓ Salmon contains omega-3 fatty acids, vitamin D, and calcium.
- ✓ Mixed veggies offer vitamins, minerals, and antioxidants.
- ✓ Olive oil provides healthful fats and antioxidants.
- ✓ Lemon: Enhances flavor and contains vitamin C.

Benefit for Osteoporosis: This grilled salmon and roasted veggie dish is high in minerals that are beneficial to bone health. Salmon contains omega-3 fatty acids and vitamin D, which improve calcium absorption and bone health. Mixed veggies contain a variety of vitamins and minerals that promote overall bone health and wellness.

Quinoa and Black Bean Stuffed Bell Peppers

Ingredients:

- 2 bell peppers, halved and seeded
- 1 cup cooked quinoa
- 1 cup black beans, drained and rinsed
- 1/2 cup diced tomatoes
- 1/4 cup diced red onion
- 1/4 cup shredded cheddar cheese

- 1 tablespoon olive oil
- 1 teaspoon ground cumin
- 1/2 teaspoon chili powder
- Salt and pepper to taste

Instructions:

1. Preheat the oven to 375° Fahrenheit (190° Celsius).
2. In a large mixing bowl, combine cooked quinoa, black beans, diced tomatoes, red onion, shredded cheddar cheese, olive oil, ground cumin, chili powder, salt, and pepper.
3. Fill each bell pepper half with the quinoa-black bean mixture.
4. Place the stuffed bell peppers in a baking dish and wrap with foil.
5. Bake the peppers in a preheated oven for 25-30 minutes, or until tender.
6. Remove the foil and bake for 5 more minutes, or until the cheese is melted and bubbling.
7. Garnish with fresh cilantro before serving.

Nutritional value:

- ✓ Quinoa is rich in protein, fiber, and minerals such as calcium and magnesium.
- ✓ Black beans include protein, fiber, and minerals that are important to bone health.
- ✓ Bell peppers are high in vitamin C, vitamin K, and antioxidants.
- ✓ Tomatoes and red onions provide vitamins, minerals, and antioxidants.
- ✓ Cheddar cheese provides calcium and taste.
- ✓ Olive oil contains heart-healthy lipids and antioxidants.

Benefits for Osteoporosis: This quinoa and black bean stuffed bell peppers recipe is a nutrient-dense, filling meal that promotes bone health. Quinoa and black beans are plant-based sources of protein and critical minerals that promote bone strength. Bell peppers include vitamin C, which promotes collagen formation and bone structure.

Baked Chicken with Sweet Potato and Broccoli

Ingredients:

- 6 oz boneless, skinless chicken breast
- 1 medium sweet potato, peeled and diced
- 1 cup broccoli florets
- 1 tablespoon olive oil
- 1 teaspoon garlic powder
- 1/2 teaspoon paprika
- Salt and pepper to taste
- Fresh parsley for garnish (optional)

Instructions:

1. Preheat the oven to 400 °F (200 °C).

2. Place the diced sweet potatoes and broccoli florets on a baking sheet. Drizzle olive oil and season with garlic powder, paprika, salt, and pepper. Toss to coat evenly.
3. Season the chicken breast with salt, pepper, and a touch of paprika.
4. Place the seasoned chicken breast on the baking pan, alongside the sweet potato and broccoli.
5. Bake in the preheated oven for 20-25 minutes, or until the chicken is fully cooked and the vegetables are soft.
6. Garnish with fresh parsley before serving.

Nutritional value:

- ✓ Chicken breast is an excellent source of lean protein and vital amino acids.
- ✓ Sweet potato is high in vitamins A, C, and potassium.
- ✓ Broccoli provides vitamin K, calcium, and fiber.
- ✓ Olive oil contains beneficial lipids and antioxidants.
- ✓ Garlic powder and paprika: Enhance flavor and provide antioxidants.

Benefits for Osteoporosis: This roasted chicken with sweet potato and broccoli is a nutritious meal that promotes bone health. Chicken breast contains the high-quality protein required to preserve bone density and muscle strength. Sweet potatoes and broccoli provide a variety of vitamins and minerals that are necessary for bone metabolism and density.

Salmon and Asparagus Foil Packets

Ingredients:

- 4 oz salmon fillet
- 1 cup asparagus spears, trimmed
- 1/2 cup cherry tomatoes, halved
- 1/4 cup sliced red onion
- 1 tablespoon olive oil
- 1 tablespoon lemon juice
- 1 teaspoon Dijon mustard
- 1/2 teaspoon dried dill
- Salt and pepper to taste

Instructions:

1. Preheat the oven to 400 °F (200 °C).
2. Place a piece of aluminum foil on a baking sheet. Place the salmon fillet, asparagus spears, cherry tomatoes, and sliced red onion on the foil.
3. In a small bowl, combine the olive oil, lemon juice, Dijon mustard, dried dill, salt, and pepper.
4. Drizzle the dressing on the fish and vegetables.
5. Fold the foil over the salmon and vegetables to form a packet, and then seal the sides tightly.
6. Bake in a preheated oven for 15-20 minutes, or until the salmon

is fully cooked and the vegetables are soft.

7. Carefully open the foil packets and serve when hot.

Nutritional value:

✓ Salmon contains omega-3 fatty acids, vitamin D, and calcium.
✓ Asparagus provides vitamin K, calcium, and fiber.
✓ Cherry tomatoes and red onions provide vitamins, minerals, and antioxidants.
✓ Olive oil contains beneficial lipids and antioxidants.
✓ Lemon juice and Dijon mustard enhance taste and acidity.

Benefits for Osteoporosis: This salmon and asparagus foil packets recipe is a nutritious and simple dinner that promotes bone health. Salmon contains omega-3 fatty acids and vitamin D, which improve calcium absorption and bone health. Asparagus provides vitamin K, which is essential for bone metabolism and density.

Baked Chicken with Sweet Potatoes and Broccoli

Ingredients:

- 6 oz chicken breast, boneless and skinless
- 1 medium sweet potato, peeled and diced
- 1 cup broccoli florets
- 1 tablespoon olive oil
- 1 teaspoon garlic powder
- 1 teaspoon paprika
- Salt and pepper to taste
- Fresh parsley for garnish (optional)

Instructions:

1. Preheat the oven to 400 °F (200 °C).
2. Season the chicken breasts with garlic powder, paprika, salt, and pepper.
3. Arrange the seasoned chicken breast on one side of a baking sheet.
4. Mix the chopped sweet potatoes and broccoli florets with olive oil, salt, and pepper.
5. Spread the sweet potatoes and broccoli on the other side of the baking sheet.
6. Bake in the preheated oven for 20-25 minutes, or until the chicken is fully cooked and the vegetables are soft.
7. Remove from the oven and allow it to rest for a few minutes before serving.
8. Garnish with fresh parsley before serving.

Nutritional value:

✓ Chicken breast is a high-quality protein source rich in phosphorus and vitamin B6.
✓ Sweet potatoes contain beta-carotene, vitamin C, and potassium.
✓ Broccoli is high in calcium, vitamin K, and antioxidants.

✓ Olive oil contains beneficial lipids and antioxidants.

Benefits for Osteoporosis: This roasted chicken with sweet potatoes and broccoli is a nutritious dinner that promotes bone health. Chicken breast provides the protein required for bone and muscle function. Sweet potatoes contain vitamin C, which aids in collagen synthesis, as well as potassium, which neutralizes acids that can deplete calcium from bones. Broccoli contains high levels of calcium, vitamin K, and antioxidants, all of which enhance bone health and density.

Spinach and Mushroom Stuffed Chicken Breast

Ingredients:

- 2 boneless, skinless chicken breasts
- 1 cup fresh spinach leaves
- 1/2 cup sliced mushrooms
- 1/4 cup shredded mozzarella cheese
- 1 tablespoon olive oil
- 1 clove garlic, minced
- Salt and pepper to taste
- Toothpicks

Instructions:

1. Preheat the oven to 375° Fahrenheit (190° Celsius).
2. In a skillet, heat the olive oil over medium heat. Add the minced garlic and cook until fragrant.
3. Cook the spinach leaves and sliced mushrooms in the skillet until they are wilted and soft. Remove from heat.
4. Butterfly each chicken breast by slicing it horizontally across the center, leaving one edge intact.
5. Open the chicken breasts and lay them between two sheets of plastic wrap. Pound them into a consistent thickness.
6. Season the insides of each chicken breast with salt and pepper.
7. Divide the spinach and mushroom mixture evenly among the chicken breasts, arranging it on one side of each.
8. Sprinkle shredded mozzarella cheese over the spinach and mushrooms.
9. Fold the other side of each chicken breast over the filling, then attach with toothpicks.
10. Bake the packed chicken breasts in a preheated oven for 25-30 minutes, or until well done.
11. Remove from the oven and allow it to rest for a few minutes before serving.

Nutritional value:

- ✓ Chicken breast: A lean protein source high in phosphorus and niacin.
- ✓ Spinach provides calcium, magnesium, and vitamin K.

- ✓ Mushrooms include vitamin D and antioxidants.
- ✓ Mozzarella cheese provides calcium and taste.
- ✓ Olive oil contains beneficial lipids and antioxidants.

Benefits for Osteoporosis: This spinach and mushroom-filled chicken breast recipe is a tasty and nutritious way to promote bone health. Spinach and mushrooms include critical vitamins and minerals that promote bone density and strength. Chicken breast contains the high-quality protein required to preserve bone mass and muscle strength.

Turkey Meatballs with Whole Wheat Pasta

Ingredients:

- 8 oz lean ground turkey
- 1/4 cup whole wheat breadcrumbs
- 1/4 cup grated Parmesan cheese
- 1 egg
- 1/4 cup chopped fresh parsley
- 1 clove garlic, minced
- 1/2 teaspoon dried oregano
- Salt and pepper to taste
- 8 oz whole wheat spaghetti
- 2 cups marinara sauce
- Fresh basil leaves for garnish (optional)

Instructions:

1. Preheat the oven to 400 °F (200 °C).
2. In a large mixing bowl, combine ground turkey, whole wheat breadcrumbs, grated Parmesan cheese, egg, chopped parsley, minced garlic, dried oregano, salt, and pepper. Mix until thoroughly mixed.
3. Shape the turkey mixture into meatballs and arrange on a baking sheet lined with parchment paper.
4. Bake in the preheated oven for 15-20 minutes, or until the meatballs are thoroughly cooked and gently browned.
5. Meanwhile, cook the whole wheat spaghetti per the package directions. Drain and set aside.
6. In a large skillet, cook the marinara sauce over medium heat.
7. Toss the cooked meatballs in the skillet with the marinara sauce until evenly coated.
8. Serve the turkey meatballs with marinara sauce over cooked whole wheat spaghetti.
9. Garnish with fresh basil leaves before serving.

Nutritional value:

- ✓ Lean ground turkey contains protein, niacin, and zinc.
- ✓ Whole wheat breadcrumbs and pasta provide fiber and important minerals.
- ✓ Parmesan cheese provides calcium and taste.
- ✓ Fresh parsley and basil provide vitamins and antioxidants.

✓ Marinara sauce contains vitamins from tomatoes and herbs.

Benefits of Osteoporosis: This turkey meatballs with whole wheat spaghetti recipe is a filling and nutrient-dense way to enhance bone health. Lean ground turkey provides the protein required for bone and muscle health. Whole wheat pasta contains fiber and important minerals that promote overall bone health. Parmesan cheese contains calcium, which is necessary for bone density and strength.

Salmon and Asparagus Sheet Pan Dinner

Ingredients:

- 2 salmon fillets
- 1 bunch asparagus, trimmed
- 2 tablespoons olive oil
- 2 cloves garlic, minced
- 1 lemon, sliced
- Salt and pepper to taste
- Fresh dill for garnish (optional)

Instructions:

1. Preheat the oven to 400 °F (200 °C).
2. Arrange the salmon fillets and trimmed asparagus on a large baking sheet.
3. Drizzle olive oil on the fish and asparagus. Sprinkle the minced garlic, salt, and pepper equally over everything.
4. Place lemon slices on top of the salmon fillets.
5. Bake in a preheated oven for 12-15 minutes, or until the salmon is fully cooked and the asparagus is soft.
6. Remove from the oven and garnish with fresh dill before serving.

Nutritional value:

- ✓ Salmon contains omega-3 fatty acids and vitamin D.
- ✓ Asparagus provides vitamin K, folate, and fiber.
- ✓ Olive oil contains beneficial lipids and antioxidants.
- ✓ Lemon: Enhances flavor and contains vitamin C.

Benefits for Osteoporosis: This salmon and asparagus sheet pan dinner is a nutritious and simple dish that promotes bone health. Salmon contains high levels of omega-3 fatty acids and vitamin D, both of which are necessary for bone density and strength. Asparagus contains vitamin K, which aids in bone metabolism and calcium absorption.

Bean and Vegetable Stir-Fry

Ingredients:

- 1 can (15 oz) mixed beans, drained and rinsed
- 2 cups mixed vegetables (bell peppers, snap peas, carrots)
- 1/4 cup diced onion
- 2 cloves garlic, minced

- 2 tablespoons low-sodium soy sauce
- 1 tablespoon olive oil
- 1 teaspoon grated ginger
- Sesame seeds for garnish

Instructions:

1. Heat the olive oil in a large skillet or wok over medium heat.
2. Sauté sliced onion and minced garlic in the skillet until fragrant.
3. Stir-fry the mixed vegetables in the skillet until they are soft and crispy.
4. Cook the mixed beans and grated ginger in the skillet until they are heated through.
5. Stir in the low-sodium soy sauce and simmer for another minute.
6. Remove from heat and sprinkle with sesame seeds before serving.

Nutritional value:

- ✓ Mixed beans offer protein, fiber, and minerals such as calcium and magnesium.
- ✓ Mixed veggies provide vitamins, minerals, and antioxidants.
- ✓ Onions and garlic contain chemicals that can protect bones.
- ✓ Low-sodium soy sauce: Enhances flavor without adding too much sodium.

- ✓ Olive oil provides healthful fats and antioxidants.

Benefits for Osteoporosis: This bean and vegetable stir-fry is a nutritious and tasty meal that promotes bone health. Mixed beans are a plant-based source of protein and critical minerals that promote bone strength. Mixed veggies contain vitamins and antioxidants that help reduce inflammation and promote bone health.

Grilled Chicken Caesar Salad

Ingredients:

- 6 oz grilled chicken breast, sliced
- 4 cups romaine lettuce, chopped
- 1/4 cup cherry tomatoes, halved
- 1/4 cup sliced cucumber
- 2 tablespoons grated Parmesan cheese
- 2 tablespoons Caesar dressing
- 1 tablespoon lemon juice
- Salt and pepper to taste
- Croutons for garnish (optional)

Instructions:

1. In a large bowl, combine chopped romaine lettuce, cherry tomatoes, sliced cucumber, and grated Parmesan cheese.
2. Add sliced grilled chicken breast to the salad.
3. In a small bowl, whisk together Caesar dressing and lemon juice.

4. Drizzle the dressing over the salad and toss to coat evenly.
5. Season with salt and pepper to taste.
6. Garnish with croutons before serving, if desired.

Nutritional Value:

- ✓ Grilled chicken breast contains lean protein and important minerals.
- ✓ Romaine lettuce contains calcium, magnesium, and vitamin K.
- ✓ Cherry tomatoes and cucumbers provide vitamins, minerals, and water.
- ✓ Parmesan cheese provides calcium and taste.
- ✓ Caesar dressing provides flavor and healthful fats.

Benefits for Osteoporosis: This grilled chicken Caesar salad is a pleasant and nutrient-dense meal that promotes bone health. Grilled chicken breast contains the protein required for bone and muscle maintenance. Romaine lettuce provides vitamin K, which is necessary for bone metabolism and calcium absorption.

Salmon and Asparagus Foil Packets

Ingredients:

- 2 salmon fillets
- 1 bunch asparagus, trimmed
- 2 tablespoons olive oil
- 2 cloves garlic, minced
- 1 lemon, sliced
- Salt and pepper to taste
- Fresh dill for garnish (optional)

Instructions:

1. Preheat the oven to 400 °F (200 °C).
2. Place each salmon fillet in the center of a wide piece of aluminum foil that may be wrapped around it.
3. Arrange the trimmed asparagus around the salmon fillets.
4. Drizzle olive oil on the fish and asparagus.
5. Sprinkle minced garlic over the fish and asparagus.
6. Season with salt and pepper to taste.
7. Put lemon wedges on top of each salmon fillet.
8. Fold the sides of the aluminum foil over the salmon and asparagus to form a package.
9. Place the foil packets on a baking sheet and bake in a preheated oven for 15-20 minutes or until the salmon and asparagus are soft.
10. Carefully unwrap the foil packs and place the fish and asparagus on plates.
11. Garnish with fresh dill before serving.

Nutritional value:

- ✓ Salmon contains omega-3 fatty acids, vitamin D, and calcium.

✓ Asparagus provides vitamin K, folate, and antioxidants.
✓ Olive oil contains beneficial lipids and antioxidants.
✓ Lemon: Enhances flavor and contains vitamin C.

Benefits for Osteoporosis: This salmon and asparagus foil packets recipe is a nutritious and simple dinner that promotes bone health. Salmon contains omega-3 fatty acids and vitamin D, which are required for calcium absorption and bone strength. Asparagus contains vitamin K, which aids bone metabolism and calcium management.

Vegetable and Tofu Stir-Fry

Ingredients:

- 8 oz firm tofu, cubed
- 2 cups mixed vegetables (bell peppers, broccoli, carrots)
- 1/4 cup sliced onion
- 2 cloves garlic, minced
- 2 tablespoons low-sodium soy sauce
- 1 tablespoon sesame oil
- 1 tablespoon rice vinegar
- 1 teaspoon grated ginger
- Sesame seeds for garnish

Instructions:

1. To remove any extra moisture, press the tofu between paper towels. Cut into cubes.
2. In a large skillet or wok, heat the sesame oil over medium heat.
3. Add the sliced onion and minced garlic to the skillet and cook until fragrant.
4. Cook the cubed tofu until it's lightly browned on all sides.
5. Stir-fry the mixed vegetables in the skillet until they are soft and crispy.
6. In a small bowl, combine the low-sodium soy sauce, rice vinegar, and grated ginger.
7. Pour the soy sauce mixture onto the tofu and vegetables in the skillet.
8. Cook for another 2-3 minutes, stirring periodically, until cooked through.
9. Remove from heat and sprinkle with sesame seeds before serving.

Nutritional value:

✓ Tofu is an excellent source of plant-based protein, calcium, and magnesium.
✓ Mixed veggies offer vitamins, minerals, and antioxidants.
✓ Onions and garlic contain chemicals that have the ability to protect bones.
✓ Low-sodium soy sauce: Enhances flavor without adding too much sodium.
✓ Sesame oil provides healthful fats and taste.

Benefit for Osteoporosis: This vegetable and tofu stir-fry is a nutrient-dense and filling meal that promotes bone health. Tofu contains plant-based protein and critical minerals that are necessary for bone strength and density. Mixed veggies contain vitamins and antioxidants that help reduce inflammation and promote bone health.

Greek Salad with Grilled Chicken

Ingredients:

- 6 oz grilled chicken breast, sliced
- 2 cups mixed salad greens (romaine lettuce, spinach, arugula)
- 1 cucumber, sliced
- 1 cup cherry tomatoes, halved
- 1/4 cup sliced red onion
- 1/4 cup Kalamata olives
- 1/4 cup crumbled feta cheese
- 2 tablespoons extra virgin olive oil
- 1 tablespoon red wine vinegar
- 1 teaspoon dried oregano
- Salt and pepper to taste

Instructions:

1. In a large bowl, combine mixed salad greens, sliced cucumber, halved cherry tomatoes, sliced red onion, Kalamata olives, and crumbled feta cheese.
2. The dressing is made by whisking together extra virgin olive oil, red wine vinegar, dried oregano, salt, and pepper in a small bowl.
3. Drizzle the dressing over the salad and toss to distribute evenly.
4. Divide the salad mixture among the serving dishes.
5. Top each salad with sliced grilled chicken breast.

Nutritional value:

- ✓ Grilled chicken breast is a healthy source of protein, niacin, and phosphorus.
- ✓ Mixed salad greens provide vitamins, minerals, and fiber.
- ✓ Cucumber with cherry tomatoes: High in vitamins and water.
- ✓ Red onion and Kalamata olives provide flavor and antioxidants.
- ✓ Feta cheese provides calcium and taste.
- ✓ Olive oil and red wine vinegar provide beneficial lipids and acidity.

Benefits for Osteoporosis: This Greek salad with grilled chicken is a pleasant and nutrient-dense meal that promotes bone health. Grilled chicken breast provides the protein required for bone and muscle preservation. Mixed salad greens contain calcium, magnesium, and vitamin K, all of which are needed for bone health and density. Feta cheese adds calcium, while olives and olive oil contain heart-healthy fats and antioxidants.

Vegetable and Lentil Stew

Ingredients:

- 1 cup dried green or brown lentils, rinsed and drained
- 4 cups vegetable broth
- 1 onion, diced
- 2 carrots, diced
- 2 celery stalks, diced
- 2 cloves garlic, minced
- 1 teaspoon ground cumin
- 1/2 teaspoon smoked paprika
- Salt and pepper to taste
- Fresh parsley for garnish (optional)

Instructions:

1. In a large pot, heat the olive oil over medium heat. Cook the diced onion, carrots, and celery until softened.
2. Cook for another minute, stirring in the minced garlic, ground cumin, and smoky paprika.
3. Add the washed lentils and vegetable broth to the pot. Bring to a boil, then reduce the heat and simmer for 20-25 minutes, or until the lentils are cooked.
4. Season the stew with salt and pepper, to taste.
5. Serve hot, topped with fresh parsley if preferred.

Nutritional value:

- ✓ Lentils are an excellent source of protein, fiber, and minerals such as calcium, magnesium, and phosphorous.
- ✓ Vegetables (onion, carrots, celery) include vitamins, minerals, and antioxidants.
- ✓ Garlic contains chemicals with possible bone-protective effects.
- ✓ Spices (cumin, paprika): They enhance flavor and may have anti-inflammatory properties.
- ✓ Fresh parsley adds freshness while also providing essential vitamins and minerals.

Benefits for Osteoporosis: This vegetable and lentil stew is a nourishing and soothing meal that promotes bone health. Lentils are a plant-based source of protein and vital minerals that promote bone health and density. Vegetables provide vitamins and antioxidants that help reduce inflammation and promote bone health.

Salmon and Quinoa Salad

Ingredients:

- 4 oz grilled salmon fillet
- 1 cup cooked quinoa
- 1 cup mixed greens (spinach, arugula, romaine)
- 1/2 cup cherry tomatoes, halved
- 1/4 cup sliced cucumber
- 2 tablespoons sliced almonds
- 2 tablespoons crumbled feta cheese
- 2 tablespoons extra virgin olive oil
- 1 tablespoon lemon juice

- Salt and pepper to taste

Instructions:

- In a large mixing bowl, add cooked quinoa, mixed greens, cherry tomatoes, sliced cucumber, almonds, and crumbled feta cheese.
- Drizzle extra virgin olive oil and lemon juice over the salad.
- Season with salt and pepper to taste.
- Toss lightly to combine all ingredients.
- Grilled salmon fillet should be placed on top of the salad.

Nutritional value:

- ✓ Salmon contains omega-3 fatty acids, vitamin D, and calcium.
- ✓ Quinoa contains protein, fiber, and minerals such as calcium and magnesium.
- ✓ Mixed greens provide calcium, magnesium, and vitamin K.
- ✓ Cherry tomatoes and cucumbers are high in vitamins and antioxidants.
- ✓ Almonds contain protein, healthy fats, and calcium.
- ✓ Feta cheese provides calcium and taste.
- ✓ Olive oil contains heart-healthy lipids and antioxidants.

Benefits for Osteoporosis: This salmon and quinoa salad is a nutritious meal that promotes bone health. Salmon contains omega-3 fatty acids and vitamin D, which improve calcium absorption and bone health. Quinoa contains plant-based protein and minerals that are needed for bone density.

Chicken and Vegetable Stir-Fry

Ingredients:

- 6 oz boneless, skinless chicken breast, sliced
- 2 cups mixed vegetables (bell peppers, broccoli, carrots)
- 1/4 cup sliced onion
- 2 cloves garlic, minced
- 2 tablespoons low-sodium soy sauce
- 1 tablespoon sesame oil
- 1 tablespoon rice vinegar
- 1 teaspoon grated ginger
- 1 teaspoon honey
- Sesame seeds for garnish

Instructions:

1. Heat the sesame oil in a large skillet over medium heat.
2. Add the sliced onion and minced garlic to the skillet and cook until fragrant.
3. Cook the sliced chicken breast in the skillet until it is browned and well done.
4. Stir-fry the mixed vegetables in the skillet until they are soft and crispy.
5. In a small bowl, combine the low-sodium soy sauce, rice vinegar, grated ginger, and honey.

6. Pour the soy sauce mixture onto the chicken and veggies in the skillet.
7. Cook for a another 2-3 minutes, stirring periodically, until cooked through.
8. Remove from heat and sprinkle with sesame seeds before serving.

Nutritional value:

- ✓ Chicken breast is a lean source of protein, vitamin B6, and niacin.
- ✓ Mixed veggies offer vitamins, minerals, and antioxidants.
- ✓ Onions and garlic contain chemicals that have the ability to protect bones.
- ✓ Low-sodium soy sauce: Enhances flavor without adding too much sodium.
- ✓ Sesame oil provides healthful fats and taste.
- ✓ Rice vinegar and ginger provide acidity and depth of flavor.

Benefit for Osteoporosis: This chicken and vegetable stir-fry is a balanced and tasty meal that promotes bone health. Chicken breast contains the protein required to maintain bone density and muscle strength. Mixed veggies contain vitamins and antioxidants that help reduce inflammation and promote bone health.

Mediterranean Chickpea Salad

Ingredients:

- 1 can (15 oz) chickpeas, drained and rinsed
- 1 cucumber, diced
- 1 cup cherry tomatoes, halved
- 1/4 cup diced red onion
- 1/4 cup chopped fresh parsley
- 2 tablespoons extra virgin olive oil
- 1 tablespoon lemon juice
- 1 teaspoon dried oregano
- Salt and pepper to taste
- Crumbled feta cheese for garnish (optional)

Instructions:

1. In a large mixing dish, combine chickpeas, diced cucumber, cherry tomatoes, diced red onion, and chopped parsley.
2. In a small bowl, combine the extra virgin olive oil, lemon juice, dried oregano, salt, and pepper.
3. Pour the dressing over the chickpea salad and stir gently.
4. If preferred, garnish with crumbled feta cheese before serving.
5. Serve chilled or at room temperature.

Nutritional value:

- ✓ Chickpeas are high in protein, fiber, and minerals like calcium, magnesium, and phosphorus.
- ✓ Cucumbers and tomatoes provide vitamins, minerals, and antioxidants.

✓ Red onion: Enhances flavor and includes chemicals with possible bone-protective effects.
✓ Olive oil contains heart-healthy lipids and antioxidants.
✓ Lemon juice and oregano add both freshness and flavor.

Benefits for Osteoporosis: This Mediterranean chickpea salad is a tasty and nutrient-dense dish that promotes bone health. Chickpeas contain plant-based proteins and critical elements that are necessary for bone strength and density. The vegetables in the salad include vitamins and antioxidants that improve bone health and overall well-being.

Tofu and Vegetable Stir-Fry

Ingredients:

- 8 oz extra-firm tofu, cubed
- 2 cups mixed vegetables (bell peppers, snap peas, carrots)
- 1/4 cup sliced mushrooms
- 2 cloves garlic, minced
- 2 tablespoons low-sodium soy sauce
- 1 tablespoon sesame oil
- 1 tablespoon rice vinegar
- 1 teaspoon grated ginger
- 1 teaspoon honey
- Sesame seeds for garnish

Instructions:

1. In a large mixing dish, combine chickpeas, diced cucumber, cherry tomatoes, diced red onion, and chopped parsley.
2. In a small bowl, combine the extra virgin olive oil, lemon juice, dried oregano, salt, and pepper.
3. Pour the dressing over the chickpea salad and stir gently.
4. If preferred, garnish with crumbled feta cheese before serving.
5. Serve chilled or at room temperature.

Nutritional value:

✓ Chickpeas are high in protein, fiber, and minerals like calcium, magnesium, and phosphorus.
✓ Cucumbers and tomatoes provide vitamins, minerals, and antioxidants.
✓ Red onion: Enhances flavor and includes chemicals with possible bone-protective effects.
✓ Olive oil contains heart-healthy lipids and antioxidants.
✓ Lemon juice and oregano add both freshness and flavor.

Benefits for Osteoporosis: This Mediterranean chickpea salad is a tasty and nutrient-dense dish that promotes bone health. Chickpeas contain plant-based proteins and critical elements that are necessary for bone strength and density. The vegetables in the salad include vitamins and antioxidants that improve bone health and overall well-being.

Turkey and Quinoa Stuffed Bell Peppers

Ingredients:

- 4 bell peppers, halved and seeded
- 1 cup cooked quinoa
- 1 lb ground turkey
- 1/2 cup diced onion
- 1/2 cup diced tomatoes
- 1/4 cup shredded mozzarella cheese
- 1 tablespoon olive oil
- 1 teaspoon dried oregano
- 1/2 teaspoon garlic powder
- Salt and pepper to taste
- Fresh parsley for garnish (optional)

Instructions:

1. Preheat the oven to 375° Fahrenheit (190° Celsius).
2. In a large skillet, heat the olive oil over medium heat. Add the diced onion and heat until softened.
3. Cook the ground turkey in the skillet until it is browned and well-cooked.
4. Stir in the cooked quinoa, diced tomatoes, dry oregano, garlic powder, salt, and pepper. Cook for another 2-3 minutes, until well heated.
5. Fill each bell pepper half with the turkey-quinoa mixture.
6. Place the stuffed bell peppers in a baking dish and wrap them in foil.
7. Bake the peppers in a preheated oven for 25-30 minutes, or until tender.
8. Remove the foil and sprinkle the filled peppers with shredded mozzarella cheese. Bake for a further 5 minutes, or until the cheese melts and bubbles.
9. Garnish with fresh parsley before serving.

Nutritional value:

- ✓ Turkey is a lean protein source rich in niacin and vitamin B6.
- ✓ Quinoa contains protein, fiber, and minerals such as calcium and magnesium.
- ✓ Bell peppers are high in vitamin C, vitamin K, and antioxidants.
- ✓ Tomatoes and onions provide vitamins, minerals, and antioxidants.
- ✓ Mozzarella cheese provides calcium and taste.
- ✓ Olive oil contains beneficial lipids and antioxidants.

Benefits for Osteoporosis: This turkey and quinoa stuffed bell peppers are a nutrient-dense and tasty choice for bone health. Turkey supplies the protein required for bone and muscle maintenance. Quinoa contains plant-based protein and critical elements that are necessary for bone density and strength.

Bell peppers include vitamin C, which promotes collagen synthesis and bone structure.

Mushroom and Spinach Stuffed Portobello Mushrooms

Ingredients:

- 4 large Portobello mushrooms, stems removed
- 2 cups fresh spinach leaves
- 1 cup diced mushrooms
- 1/4 cup diced onion
- 2 cloves garlic, minced
- 1/4 cup shredded mozzarella cheese
- 2 tablespoons grated Parmesan cheese
- 1 tablespoon olive oil
- Salt and pepper to taste
- Fresh parsley for garnish (optional)

Instructions:

1. Preheat the oven to 375° Fahrenheit (190° Celsius). Line a baking sheet with parchment paper.
2. Place the Portobello mushrooms on the baking sheet, gills facing up.
3. In a skillet, heat the olive oil over medium heat. Sauté diced onion and minced garlic until aromatic.
4. Cook the diced mushrooms in the skillet until they soften.
5. Cook the fresh spinach leaves in the skillet until wilted.
6. Remove the skillet from the heat and add the shredded mozzarella cheese, stirring until melted.
7. Season the spinach and mushroom mixture with salt and pepper, to taste.
8. Spoon the spinach and mushroom mixture into the hollow of each Portobello mushroom.
9. Sprinkle-grated Parmesan cheese over the filled mushrooms.
10. Bake in a preheated oven for 15-20 minutes, or until the mushrooms are soft and the cheese is melted and bubbling.
11. Remove from the oven and allow it to cool for a few minutes before serving.
12. Garnish with fresh parsley before serving.

Nutritional value:

- ✓ Portobello mushrooms include vitamin D and minerals such as selenium and potassium.
- ✓ Spinach is high in calcium, magnesium, and vitamin K.
- ✓ Mushrooms include vitamin D and antioxidants.
- ✓ Mozzarella and Parmesan cheeses provide calcium and taste.
- ✓ Olive oil contains beneficial lipids and antioxidants.

Benefits for Osteoporosis: This mushroom and spinach stuffed Portobello mushroom recipe is a delightful and nutrient-dense way to enhance bone health. Portobello mushrooms contain vitamin D, which promotes calcium absorption and bone metabolism. Spinach contains calcium and vitamin K, which are needed for bone density and strength. The mix of mushrooms and cheese adds calcium and flavor to the dish, making it a filling and bone-friendly option.

CHAPTER 5: SNACKS FOR BONE HEALTH RECIPES

Greek Yogurt Parfait with Berries and Almonds

Ingredients:

- 1 cup Greek yogurt
- 1/2 cup mixed berries (strawberries, blueberries, raspberries)
- 2 tablespoons sliced almonds
- 1 tablespoon honey (optional)

Instructions:

1. In a small bowl or glass, combine the Greek yogurt, mixed berries, and chopped almonds.
2. Repeat the layering until all ingredients have been utilized.
3. If desired, drizzle honey over the top to add sweetness.
4. Serve immediately, or chill until ready to eat.

Nutritional value:

- ✓ Greek yogurt is high in protein and calcium, which are needed for bone health.
- ✓ Mixed berries are high in antioxidants and vitamin C, which promotes collagen formation.
- ✓ Almonds include calcium, magnesium, and vitamin E, which are all advantageous to bone density.
- ✓ Honey provides sweetness and contains trace levels of minerals such as manganese and copper.

Benefits for Osteoporosis: This Greek yogurt parfait with berries and almonds is a healthy and enjoyable snack that promotes bone health. Greek yogurt contains a high concentration of protein and calcium, both of which are essential for bone health. Berries include antioxidants, which help reduce inflammation and preserve bone cells from injury. Almonds include calcium and magnesium, two minerals that are essential for bone density and structure.

Cottage Cheese and Veggie Dip

Ingredients:

- 1/2 cup low-fat cottage cheese
- 1/4 cup diced bell peppers (red, yellow, green)
- 1/4 cup diced cucumber
- 2 tablespoons chopped carrots
- 1 tablespoon chopped fresh parsley
- 1/2 teaspoon garlic powder
- Salt and pepper to taste
- Baby carrots and cucumber slices for dipping

Instructions:

1. Mix cottage cheese in a blender or food processor until smooth.
2. Place the blended cottage cheese in a bowl.
3. Add diced bell peppers, cucumber, carrots, chopped parsley, garlic powder, salt, and pepper, and mix thoroughly.
4. Serve the cottage cheese and vegetable dip with baby carrots and cucumber slices for dipping.

Nutritional Value:

- ✓ Cottage cheese is a high-protein, calcium-rich food that is important for bone health.
- ✓ Bell peppers include vitamin C, which assists collagen synthesis and promotes bone structure.
- ✓ Cucumbers and carrots are high in vitamins, minerals, and antioxidants, which help to maintain bone health.
- ✓ Fresh parsley: Enhances flavor and includes vitamin K, which is essential for bone mineralization.

Benefits for Osteoporosis: This cottage cheese and veggie dip is a healthy and quick snack that promotes bone health. Cottage cheese has high levels of protein and calcium, both of which are essential for bone density and muscular function. The combination of bell peppers, cucumbers, and carrots contains vitamins and minerals that promote bone health and wellness.

Spinach and Feta Stuffed Mini Bell Peppers

Ingredients:

- 10 mini bell peppers, halved and seeds removed
- 1 cup fresh spinach, chopped
- 1/4 cup crumbled feta cheese
- 2 tablespoons diced red onion
- 1 clove garlic, minced
- 1 tablespoon olive oil
- Salt and pepper to taste

Instructions:

1. Preheat oven to 375°F (190°C). Line a baking sheet with parchment paper.

2. In a skillet, heat olive oil over medium heat. Sauté sliced red onion and minced garlic until tender.

3. Cook chopped spinach in skillet until wilted. Remove from heat.

4. Mix in crumbled feta cheese until thoroughly mixed. Season with salt and pepper to taste.

5. Spoon spinach and feta mixture into halved tiny bell peppers.

6. Arrange stuffed small bell peppers on a prepared baking sheet.

7. Bake for 12-15 minutes in a preheated oven until the peppers are

soft and the filling is thoroughly cooked.

8. Allow it to cool for a few minutes before serving.

Nutritional value:

- ✓ Mini bell peppers include vitamin C and antioxidants.
- ✓ Spinach is high in calcium, magnesium, and vitamin K.
- ✓ Feta cheese provides calcium and taste.
- ✓ Red onion and garlic include chemicals that can protect bones.
- ✓ Olive oil contains beneficial lipids and antioxidants.

Benefits for Osteoporosis: These spinach and feta stuffed tiny bell peppers are a delightful, nutrient-dense snack that promotes bone health. Spinach contains calcium and vitamin K, which are needed for bone density and strength. Feta cheese provides calcium and protein to the snack, which promotes bone health and muscular performance. Mini bell peppers include vitamin C, which promotes collagen formation and bone structure.

Homemade Trail Mix with Nuts and Seeds

Ingredients:

- 1/2 cup almonds
- 1/2 cup walnuts
- 1/4 cup pumpkin seeds
- 1/4 cup sunflower seeds
- 1/4 cup dried cranberries
- 1/4 cup dark chocolate chips (optional)

Instructions:

1. In a large mixing bowl, combine almonds, walnuts, pumpkin seeds, sunflower seeds, dried cranberries, and dark chocolate chips (if using).
2. Mix thoroughly until all components are uniformly distributed.
3. Keep the homemade trail mix in an airtight container or separate it into individual snack bags for convenient grab-and-go options.

Nutritional value:

- ✓ Almonds and walnuts include calcium, magnesium, and healthful fats.
- ✓ Pumpkin seeds and sunflower seeds include protein, fiber, and minerals such as magnesium and phosphorus.
- ✓ Dried cranberries include antioxidants and vitamins.
- ✓ Dark chocolate chips are both flavorful and antioxidant-rich.

Benefits for Osteoporosis: This homemade trail mix with nuts and seeds is a simple and nutrient-dense snack that promotes bone health. Almonds, walnuts, pumpkin seeds, and sunflower seeds are high in calcium, magnesium, and other minerals required for bone strength. Dried cranberries and dark chocolate chips enhance flavor while also providing minerals and antioxidants that promote overall bone health.

Avocado and Tomato Bruschetta

Ingredients:

- 1 ripe avocado
- 1 large tomato, diced
- 2 tablespoons chopped fresh basil
- 1 tablespoon extra-virgin olive oil
- 1 teaspoon balsamic vinegar
- Salt and pepper to taste
- Slices of whole grain baguette, toasted

Instructions:

1. In a medium bowl, mash the ripe avocado until smooth.
2. Mix in sliced tomato, chopped fresh basil, extra virgin olive oil, and balsamic vinegar to the mashed avocado.
3. Season to taste with salt and pepper, then blend thoroughly.
4. Spread the avocado and tomato mixture on toasted pieces of whole-grain bread.

Nutritional value:

- ✓ Avocado contains healthful lipids, potassium, and vitamin K.
- ✓ Tomato is high in vitamin C, potassium, and antioxidants.
- ✓ Basil contains vitamin K and antioxidants.
- ✓ Extra virgin olive oil provides heart-healthy lipids and antioxidants.
- ✓ Whole grain baguette provides fiber and important minerals.

Benefits for Osteoporosis: This avocado and tomato bruschetta is a tasty, nutrient-dense snack that promotes bone health. Avocado contains healthy lipids and potassium, which help to regulate bone metabolism and maintain bone density. Tomatoes include vitamin C, which aids in collagen synthesis, and antioxidants, which protect bone cells from injury. Whole grain baguette provides fiber and important minerals that promote bone health and well-being.

Kale Chips

Ingredients:

- 4 cups kale leaves, washed and torn into bite-sized pieces
- 1 tablespoon olive oil
- 1/2 teaspoon garlic powder
- 1/2 teaspoon paprika
- Salt to taste

Instructions:

1. Preheat the oven to 350° Fahrenheit (175° Celsius).

2. In a large mixing bowl, toss the kale leaves with olive oil until thoroughly coated.
3. Toss the kale leaves with garlic powder, paprika, and salt until coated.
4. Place the seasoned kale leaves in a single layer on a baking sheet lined with parchment paper.
5. Bake the kale chips in a preheated oven for 10-15 minutes, or until crispy and lightly browned.
6. Remove from the oven and allow cooling before serving.

Nutritional value:

- ✓ Kale is high in calcium, vitamin K, and antioxidants.
- ✓ Olive oil contains beneficial lipids and antioxidants.
- ✓ Garlic powder and paprika: Enhance taste without adding too much sodium.

Benefits for Osteoporosis: Kale chips are a crispy, healthy snack that promotes bone health. Kale contains high levels of calcium and vitamin K, both of which are necessary for bone density and strength. Olive oil contains beneficial lipids that help the absorption of fat-soluble vitamins, including vitamin K.

Chia Seed Pudding

Ingredients:

- 1/4 cup chia seeds
- 1 cup unsweetened almond milk (or any milk of choice)
- 1 tablespoon maple syrup or honey
- 1/2 teaspoon vanilla extract
- Fresh fruit for topping (e.g., berries, sliced banana)

Instructions:

1. In a bowl or jar, blend the chia seeds, almond milk, maple syrup (or honey), and vanilla essence.
2. Refrigerate the dish or jar for at least 2 hours, preferably overnight, to allow the chia seeds to absorb and thicken the liquid.
3. Before serving, stir the chia seed mixture to ensure it has a uniform consistency.
4. Before serving, top with fresh fruit.

Nutritional value:

- ✓ Chia seeds contain calcium, magnesium, phosphorus, and omega-3 fatty acids.
- ✓ Almond milk has extra calcium and vitamin D.
- ✓ Maple syrup or honey: Provides sweetness without using refined sugar.
- ✓ Fresh fruit provides vitamins, minerals, and antioxidants.

Benefits for Osteoporosis: Chia seed pudding is a nutrient-dense food that promotes bone health. Chia seeds are a plant-based source of calcium, magnesium, and phosphorus, three minerals required for bone strength. Almond milk contains additional calcium and vitamin D, which are essential elements for bone density and structure.

Edamame Hummus with Veggie Sticks

Ingredients:

- 1 cup shelled edamame (cooked and cooled)
- 1/4 cup tahini
- 2 tablespoons lemon juice
- 1 clove garlic, minced
- 1/2 teaspoon ground cumin
- Salt and pepper to taste
- Baby carrots, cucumber slices, and bell pepper strips for dipping

Instructions:

1. In a food processor, combine the shelled edamame, tahini, lemon juice, minced garlic, ground cumin, salt, and pepper.
2. Process until smooth, scraping down the edges as necessary.
3. If the hummus is too thick, add a little water or olive oil to achieve the appropriate consistency.
4. Add the edamame hummus to a serving bowl.
5. Dipping options include tiny carrots, cucumber slices, and bell pepper strips.

Nutritional value:

- ✓ Edamame is an excellent source of protein, calcium, and magnesium.
- ✓ Tahini provides calcium, healthy fats, and protein.
- ✓ Lemon juice provides vitamin C and taste.
- ✓ Garlic and cumin: Enhance flavor and offer potential health advantages.

Benefits for Osteoporosis: Edamame hummus with vegetable sticks is a tasty and nutritious snack that promotes bone health. Edamame contains high levels of calcium, magnesium, and protein, all of which are necessary for bone density and strength. Tahini contains calcium and good lipids, which promote general bone health and well-being.

Cottage Cheese and Fruit Bowl

Ingredients:

- 1/2 cup low-fat cottage cheese
- 1/2 cup sliced strawberries
- 1/2 cup diced pineapple
- 1/4 cup blueberries
- 1 tablespoon chopped walnuts or almonds (optional)
- 1 teaspoon honey (optional)

Instructions:

1. In a mixing dish, combine low-fat cottage cheese.
2. Garnish with sliced strawberries, diced pineapple, and blueberries.

3. If desired, sprinkle the top with chopped walnuts or almonds.
4. If desired, drizzle with honey for an extra sweet finish.

Nutritional value:

- ✓ Cottage cheese is high in protein and calcium, which are needed for bone health.
- ✓ Strawberries, pineapple, and blueberries are high in vitamin C, antioxidants, and other minerals that promote bone health.
- ✓ Walnuts or almonds contain nutritious fats, protein, and minerals such as calcium and magnesium.
- ✓ Honey provides natural sweetness and contains trace levels of minerals.

Benefits for Osteoporosis: This cottage cheese and fruit bowl is a nutritious snack that promotes bone health. Cottage cheese contains the protein and calcium required to maintain bone density and muscular function. Fruits like strawberries, pineapple, and blueberries contain vitamin C, which aids in collagen synthesis and bone formation. Nuts such as walnuts and almonds provide calcium and magnesium, which are essential nutrients for bone health.

Avocado and Tomato Toast

Ingredients:

- 2 slices whole grain bread, toasted
- 1 ripe avocado, mashed
- 1 medium tomato, sliced
- 1 tablespoon chopped fresh basil
- 1 teaspoon lemon juice
- Salt and pepper to taste

Instructions:

1. In a mixing dish, mash the ripe avocado, then add the chopped fresh basil and lemon juice.
2. Spread the mashed avocado mixture evenly across the toasted whole-grain bread slices.
3. Top each slice with sliced tomatoes.
4. Season with salt and pepper to taste.

Nutritional value:

- ✓ Whole grain bread contains fiber, vitamins, and minerals that are needed for bone health.
- ✓ Avocado is high in healthy fats, potassium, and vitamin K, which promotes bone density and strength.
- ✓ Tomatoes provide vitamin C, antioxidants, and other minerals that promote bone health.
- ✓ Fresh basil: Adds taste and provides vitamin K, which is essential for bone mineralization.
- ✓ Lemon juice: Enhances acidity and taste.

Benefits for Osteoporosis: This avocado and tomato toast is a tasty and nutritious snack that promotes bone health. Avocados include healthful lipids and vitamin K, which are required for calcium absorption and bone metabolism. Tomatoes include vitamin C, which promotes collagen formation and bone structure. Whole grain bread contains fiber and minerals that improve bone health and wellness.

CHAPTER 6: JUICE AND SMOOTHIE RECIPES

Dear Readers,

As an author passionate about promoting health and well-being among seniors, I am thrilled to share my latest creation with you - the "Osteoporosis Diet Cookbook for Seniors." Crafting this cookbook has been a labor of love, and my ultimate goal is to empower you with delicious and nutritious recipes tailored to support your bone health journey.

Your feedback is incredibly valuable to me. As you explore the recipes and delve into the wealth of information provided, I kindly ask for your honest reviews on Amazon. Your reviews not only help me understand how the cookbook has resonated with you but also assist other seniors in making informed decisions about their health.

Whether you found a particular recipe especially delightful, discovered a helpful tip, or simply enjoyed the overall experience of using the cookbook, your thoughts matter. Your reviews not only motivate me to continue creating content that serves your needs but also contribute to building a supportive community dedicated to embracing a healthy lifestyle.

Thank you for considering sharing your thoughts with me and fellow readers. Your feedback fuels my passion for spreading knowledge and inspiration for healthier living among seniors.

Warm regards,

Green Kale and Orange Juice

Ingredients:

- 2 cups kale leaves, washed and stems removed
- 2 oranges, peeled and segmented
- 1/2 lemon, peeled and seeded
- 1 inch fresh ginger, peeled
- 1/2 cup water (optional, for desired consistency)

Instructions:

1. Combine kale leaves, orange segments, lemon, and ginger in a juicer.
2. Juice until all ingredients is thoroughly mixed and smooth.
3. If the juice is too thick, add water until it reaches the appropriate consistency.
4. Pour the juice into cups and serve immediately.

Nutritional value:

- ✓ Kale: High in calcium, vitamin K, and antioxidants, which promote bone health.
- ✓ Oranges contain vitamin C, which promotes collagen formation and calcium absorption.
- ✓ Lemon adds vitamin C and taste to the juice.
- ✓ Ginger has anti-inflammatory qualities and provides a spicy kick to the drink.
- ✓ Water helps to modify the consistency of the juice.

Benefits for Osteoporosis: This green kale and orange juice is rich in minerals that promote bone health. Kale contains high levels of calcium and vitamin K, both of which are necessary for bone density and strength. Oranges contain vitamin C, which promotes collagen formation and bone health. Ginger provides anti-inflammatory properties, which may help minimize the risk of bone loss caused by inflammation.

Berry Banana Spinach Smoothie

Ingredients:

1. 1 ripe banana
2. 1 cup fresh spinach leaves
3. 1/2 cup mixed berries (strawberries, blueberries, raspberries)
4. 1/2 cup low-fat Greek yogurt
5. 1/2 cup unsweetened almond milk (or any milk of choice)
6. 1 tablespoon chia seeds (optional)

Instructions:

1. In a blender, combine banana, spinach leaves, mixed berries, Greek yogurt, and almond milk.
2. Blend until smooth and creamy.
3. If preferred, add chia seeds and process for a few seconds to combine.
4. Pour the smoothie into cups and serve immediately.

Nutritional value:

- ✓ Banana contains potassium and vitamin B6, which are vital for bone health and metabolism.
- ✓ Spinach is high in calcium, magnesium, and vitamin K, which promote bone density and strength.
- ✓ Berries contain antioxidants and vitamin C, which are excellent for collagen formation and bone health.
- ✓ Greek yogurt is high in protein and calcium, which helps to preserve bone mass.
- ✓ Almond milk contains extra calcium and vitamin D, which are beneficial to bone health.
- ✓ Chia seeds are high in calcium, omega-3 fatty acids, and fiber, which promote bone health and digestion.

Benefits for Osteoporosis: This berry banana spinach smoothie is a tasty and nutrient-dense choice for improving bone health. Spinach, berries, and bananas include critical vitamins, minerals, and antioxidants that promote bone density and strength. Greek yogurt and almond milk include protein and calcium, which are essential for preserving bone mass and structure. Chia seeds include calcium, omega-3 fatty acids, and fiber, which improve bone health and well-being.

Tropical Mango and Pineapple Smoothie

Ingredients:

- 1 cup frozen mango chunks
- 1/2 cup fresh pineapple chunks
- 1/2 banana
- 1/2 cup low-fat Greek yogurt
- 1/2 cup coconut water
- 1 tablespoon flaxseeds (optional)

Instructions:

1. Combine frozen mango chunks, pineapple chunks, banana, Greek yogurt, and coconut water in a blender.
2. Blend until smooth and creamy.
3. If preferred, add flaxseeds and blend for a few seconds to combine.
4. Pour the smoothie into cups and serve immediately.

Nutritional value:

- ✓ Mango: High in vitamins C and A, which promote collagen formation and bone health.
- ✓ Pineapple contains vitamin C and manganese, which are crucial for bone health and metabolism.
- ✓ Bananas: Provide potassium and vitamin B6, which are good for bone density and strength.
- ✓ Greek yogurt is high in protein and calcium, both of which are needed for bone mass maintenance.
- ✓ Coconut water contains electrolytes such as potassium and magnesium, which promote bone health and hydration.

✓ Flaxseeds: High in omega-3 fatty acids and fiber, which promote bone health and digestion.

Benefits for Osteoporosis: This tropical mango and pineapple smoothie is a delicious and nutrient-dense way to promote bone health. Mango and pineapple provide vitamins and minerals that promote collagen synthesis and bone health. Greek yogurt contains protein and calcium, which are essential for preserving bone mass and structure. Coconut water contains electrolytes that help with hydration and mineral balance, which is vital for bone health.

Berry Spinach Flaxseed Smoothie

Ingredients:

- 1 cup fresh spinach leaves
- 1/2 cup mixed berries (strawberries, blueberries, raspberries)
- 1/2 banana
- 1/2 cup unsweetened almond milk (or any milk of choice)
- 1 tablespoon flaxseeds
- 1 teaspoon honey (optional)

Instructions:

1. Place spinach leaves, mixed berries, banana, almond milk, and flaxseeds in a blender.
2. Blend until smooth and creamy.
3. If desired, add honey for sweetness and blend for a few seconds to incorporate.
4. Pour the smoothie into glasses and serve immediately.

Nutritional Value:

- ✓ Spinach: Rich in calcium, magnesium, and vitamin K, which support bone density and strength.
- ✓ Berries: Provide antioxidants and vitamin C, beneficial for collagen synthesis and bone health.
- ✓ Banana: Offers potassium and vitamin B6, important for bone health and metabolism.
- ✓ Almond milk: Provides calcium and vitamin D, essential for maintaining bone mass.
- ✓ Flaxseeds: Rich in omega-3 fatty acids and fiber, which contribute to bone health and digestion.
- ✓ Honey: Adds sweetness and contains trace amounts of minerals.

Benefit for Osteoporosis: This berry spinach flaxseed smoothie is a nutrient-rich and delicious option for supporting bone health. Spinach and berries offer essential vitamins, minerals, and antioxidants that promote bone density and strength. Almond milk provides calcium and vitamin D, crucial for maintaining bone mass and structure. Flaxseeds add omega-3 fatty acids and fiber, contributing to overall bone health and digestion.

Banana and Almond Butter Smoothie

Ingredients:

- 1 ripe banana
- 2 tablespoons almond butter
- 1 cup unsweetened almond milk (or any milk of choice)
- 1/2 teaspoon ground cinnamon
- 1/2 teaspoon vanilla extract
- Ice cubes (optional)

Instructions:

1. Place ripe banana, almond butter, almond milk, ground cinnamon, vanilla extract, and ice cubes (if using) in a blender.
2. Blend until smooth and creamy.
3. Pour the smoothie into glasses and serve immediately.

Nutritional Value:

- ✓ Banana: Provides potassium and vitamin B6, essential for bone health and metabolism.
- ✓ Almond butter: Rich in calcium, magnesium, and vitamin E, which support bone density and strength.
- ✓ Almond milk: Offers calcium and vitamin D, important for maintaining bone mass.
- ✓ Cinnamon: Contains antioxidants and anti-inflammatory properties.
- ✓ Vanilla extract: Add flavor without additional calories.

Benefit for Osteoporosis: This banana and almond butter smoothie is a creamy and nutritious option for promoting bone health. Banana provides potassium, which helps regulate calcium excretion and supports bone metabolism. Almond butter offers calcium, magnesium, and vitamin E, crucial for maintaining bone density and structure.

Almond milk provides additional calcium and vitamin D, essential nutrients for bone health.

Pomegranate Berry Blast Smoothie

Ingredients:

- 1/2 cup pomegranate seeds
- 1/2 cup mixed berries (blueberries, raspberries, blackberries)
- 1/2 cup low-fat Greek yogurt
- 1/2 cup unsweetened almond milk (or any milk of choice)
- 1 tablespoon honey (optional)
- Ice cubes (optional)

Instructions:

1. Combine pomegranate seeds, mixed berries, Greek yogurt, almond milk, honey (if using), and ice cubes in a blender.
2. Blend until smooth and creamy.
3. Pour the smoothie into cups and serve immediately.

Nutritional value:

- ✓ Pomegranate seeds are high in antioxidants and vitamin C, which promote bone health and reduce inflammation.
- ✓ Mixed berries: Rich in antioxidants, vitamins, and minerals that promote bone density and strength.
- ✓ Greek yogurt is high in protein and calcium, both of which are needed for bone mass maintenance.
- ✓ Almond milk contains calcium and vitamin D, which are necessary for bone health.
- ✓ Honey: Provides sweetness without using refined sugar.

Benefits for Osteoporosis: This pomegranate berry blast smoothie is a tasty and antioxidant-rich way to promote bone health. Pomegranate seeds and mixed berries include vital elements that promote collagen formation and bone health. Greek yogurt contains protein and calcium, which are essential for maintaining bone density and structure. Almond milk contains added calcium and vitamin D, which are necessary for bone health.

Carrot Orange Ginger Juice

Ingredients:

- 3 large carrots, washed and peeled
- 2 oranges, peeled and segmented
- 1-inch piece fresh ginger, peeled
- 1/2 lemon, peeled and seeded
- Ice cubes (optional)

Instructions:

1. Pass carrots, oranges, ginger, and lemon through a juicer.
2. Once juiced, mix thoroughly to blend.
3. Pour the juice into glasses with ice cubes if desired.

Nutritional Value:

- ✓ Carrots are high in vitamins A, C, and potassium, all of which are necessary for bone health and immunological function.
- ✓ Oranges contain vitamin C, which promotes collagen formation and calcium absorption.
- ✓ Ginger has anti-inflammatory qualities and provides a spicy kick to the drink.
- ✓ Lemon adds vitamin C and taste to the juice.

Benefits for Osteoporosis: This carrot-orange ginger juice is a delicious and nutrient-dense choice for bone health. Carrots and oranges are critical vitamins and minerals promoting collagen formation and bone health. Ginger provides anti-inflammatory properties, which may help minimize the risk of bone loss caused by inflammation. Lemon contains vitamin C, which promotes bone health and the absorption of minerals such as calcium.

Spinach Banana Protein Smoothie

Ingredients:

- 1 cup fresh spinach leaves
- 1 ripe banana
- 1/2 cup low-fat Greek yogurt
- 1/2 cup unsweetened almond milk (or any milk of choice)
- 1 scoop vanilla protein powder
- 1 tablespoon almond butter
- Ice cubes (optional)

Instructions:

1. In a blender, combine spinach leaves, banana, Greek yogurt, almond milk, protein powder, almond butter, and ice cubes (if desired).
2. Blend until smooth and creamy.
3. Pour the smoothie into cups and serve immediately.

Nutritional value:

- ✓ Spinach is high in calcium, magnesium, and vitamin K, which promote bone density and strength.
- ✓ Banana contains potassium and vitamin B6, which are vital for bone health and metabolism.
- ✓ Greek yogurt is high in protein and calcium, which helps to preserve bone mass.
- ✓ Almond milk: Provides calcium and vitamin D essential for bone health.
- ✓ Protein powder: Adds protein to help maintain muscle and bone health.
- ✓ Almond butter is high in calcium, magnesium, and vitamin E, which promote bone density and structure.

Benefits for Osteoporosis: This spinach banana protein smoothie is a nutrient-dense and pleasant way to improve bone health. Spinach contains vital vitamins, minerals, and antioxidants that promote bone health and well-being. Greek yogurt contains protein and calcium, which are essential for maintaining bone mass and strength. Almond milk has more calcium and vitamin D, which are important elements for bone health.

Carrot-Orange-Ginger Juice

Ingredients:

- 4 medium carrots, washed and trimmed
- 2 oranges, peeled and segmented
- 1-inch piece of fresh ginger, peeled
- 1/2 cup water (optional, for desired consistency)
- Ice cubes (optional)

Instructions:

1. Pass carrots, oranges, and ginger through a juicer.
2. If the juice is too thick, add water to achieve the desired consistency.

3. Serve immediately over ice cubes if desired.

Nutritional Value:

- ✓ Carrots include vitamin A, which is vital for bone health and vision.
- ✓ Oranges contain vitamin C, which promotes collagen formation and bone strength.
- ✓ Ginger contains anti-inflammatory qualities that may improve bone health.
- ✓ Water helps to alter the juice's consistency without diminishing its nutrients.

Benefit for Osteoporosis: This carrot-orange-ginger juice is high in vitamins and antioxidants, which improve bone health. Carrots include beta-carotene, which the body transforms into vitamin A, which is essential for bone growth and development. Oranges contain vitamin C, which promotes collagen formation and calcium absorption. Ginger includes gingerol, which has anti-inflammatory properties and may lower the incidence of osteoporosis.

Berry-Oatmeal Smoothie

Ingredients:

- 1/2 cup mixed berries (strawberries, blueberries, raspberries)
- 1/4 cup rolled oats
- 1 ripe banana
- 1/2 cup low-fat Greek yogurt
- 1/2 cup unsweetened almond milk (or any milk of choice)
- 1 tablespoon honey (optional)
- Ice cubes (optional)

Instructions:

1. Combine mixed berries, rolled oats, banana, Greek yogurt, almond milk, honey (if using), and ice cubes (if using) in a blender.
2. Blend until smooth and creamy.
3. Pour into glasses and serve immediately.

Nutritional Value:

- ✓ Mixed berries are high in antioxidants and vitamin C, which promote bone health and prevent inflammation.
- ✓ Rolled oats provide fiber and minerals such as magnesium and phosphorus, which are beneficial to bone density.
- ✓ Banana contains potassium, which promotes bone health and regulates calcium levels.
- ✓ Greek yogurt is high in protein and calcium, which are needed for bone strength and structure.
- ✓ Almond milk contains calcium and vitamin D necessary for bone health.

Benefits for Osteoporosis: This berry-oatmeal smoothie is a nutrient-dense choice for bone health. Mixed berries contain antioxidants that prevent bone loss and promote collagen formation. Rolled oats provide fiber and minerals, which enhance bone density and overall wellness. Greek yogurt and almond milk include protein and calcium, which are essential nutrients for bone health and osteoporosis prevention.

CHAPTER 7: DESSERTS FOR BONE HEALTH RECIPES

Greek Yogurt Parfait with Nuts and Berries

Ingredients:

- 1 cup low-fat Greek yogurt
- 1/4 cup mixed nuts (almonds, walnuts, pistachios), chopped
- 1/4 cup mixed berries (strawberries, blueberries, raspberries)
- 1 tablespoon honey or maple syrup (optional)

Instructions:

1. In a glass or bowl, combine Greek yogurt, mixed almonds, and mixed berries.
2. Repeat the layering until all ingredients have been utilized.
3. For more richness, drizzle honey or maple syrup over the top.

Nutritional value:

- ✓ Greek yogurt is high in protein and calcium, which are needed for bone health.
- ✓ Mixed nuts include beneficial fats, proteins, and minerals such as calcium and magnesium.
- ✓ Mixed berries are high in antioxidants and vitamin C, which promote collagen formation and bone health.
- ✓ Honey or maple syrup: Provides natural sweetness without using processed sugar.

Benefits for Osteoporosis: This Greek yogurt parfait with nuts and berries is a delightful meal that promotes bone health. Greek yogurt is high in protein and calcium, which are required for bone density and strength. Mixed nuts provide healthful fats and minerals such as calcium and magnesium, which are essential for bone health. Mixed berries contain antioxidants that help prevent bone loss and enhance overall bone health.

Chocolate Avocado Mousse

Ingredients:

- 2 ripe avocados
- 1/4 cup cocoa powder
- 1/4 cup honey or maple syrup
- 1 teaspoon vanilla extract
- Pinch of salt
- Fresh berries for garnish (optional)

Instructions:

1. Cut the avocados in halves, remove the pits, and transfer the flesh to a blender or food processor.
2. Add the cocoa powder, honey or maple syrup, vanilla essence, and a bit of salt to the blender.
3. Blend until smooth and creamy, scraping down the sides as necessary.
4. Taste and adjust the sweetness as needed by adding more honey or maple syrup.
5. Transfer the chocolate avocado mousse to serving bowls or glasses.
6. Place in the fridge for at least 30 minutes before serving.
7. Garnish with fresh berries before serving.

Nutritional value:

- ✓ Avocado contains healthy lipids, potassium, and vitamin K, all of which are beneficial to bone health.
- ✓ Cocoa powder is high in antioxidants and flavonoids, which may aid increase bone density.
- ✓ Honey or maple syrup: Provides sweetness without using refined sugar.
- ✓ Vanilla extract enhances flavor without adding calories.
- ✓ Fresh berries provide additional antioxidants and vitamins for overall wellness.

Benefits for Osteoporosis: This chocolate avocado mousse is a delicious dessert that promotes bone health.

Avocado contains healthful lipids and potassium, which help to preserve bone density and strength. Cocoa powder includes flavonoids, which may benefit bone health by lowering inflammation and oxidative stress.

This dessert's lack of refined sugar makes it a healthier choice for those worried about bone health and overall well-being.

Chia Seed Pudding with Almond Milk and Berries

Ingredients:

- 1/4 cup chia seeds
- 1 cup unsweetened almond milk (or any milk of choice)
- 1 tablespoon honey or maple syrup
- 1/2 teaspoon vanilla extract
- 1/2 cup mixed berries (strawberries, blueberries, raspberries)

Instructions:

1. In a mixing dish, combine the chia seeds, almond milk, honey

or maple syrup, and vanilla extract.

2. To let the chia seeds to absorb and thicken, cover the bowl and refrigerate for at least 2 hours, preferably overnight.
3. Before serving, stir the chia seed mixture to ensure it has a uniform consistency.
4. Serve the chia seed pudding in individual dishes or glasses, garnished with mixed berries.

Nutritional value:

- ✓ Chia seeds are high in calcium, magnesium, phosphorus, and omega-3 fatty acids, all of which are beneficial to bone health.
- ✓ Almond milk contains calcium and vitamin D, which are essential for maintaining bone density.
- ✓ Honey or maple syrup: Provides sweetness without using refined sugar.
- ✓ Vanilla extract enhances flavor without adding calories.
- ✓ Mixed berries contain antioxidants and vitamin C, which are excellent for collagen formation and bone health.

Benefits for Osteoporosis: This chia seed pudding with almond milk and berries is a tasty and nutritious dessert that promotes bone health. Chia seeds have high levels of calcium, magnesium, and phosphorus, which are essential nutrients for bone density and strength. Almond milk has more calcium and vitamin D, both of which are necessary for bone mass maintenance. Berries include antioxidants that prevent bone loss and promote general bone health.

Baked Apples with Cinnamon and Almonds

Ingredients:

- 2 apples, cored and halved
- 1 tablespoon lemon juice
- 1 tablespoon honey or maple syrup
- 1/2 teaspoon ground cinnamon
- 2 tablespoons chopped almonds

Instructions:

1. Preheat the oven to 375° Fahrenheit (190° Celsius).
2. Put the apple halves in a baking dish and sprinkle with lemon juice.
3. In a small bowl, combine honey or maple syrup and ground cinnamon.
4. Brush the honey and cinnamon mixture over the apple halves.
5. Sprinkle chopped almonds on top of each apple half.
6. Bake in the preheated oven for 20-25 minutes, or until the apples are soft.
7. Serve the baked apples warm, with a dollop of Greek yogurt or a sprinkling of granola.

Nutritional value:

✓ Apples provide dietary fiber and vitamin C, which are essential for bone health and overall well-being.
✓ Lemon juice: Provides acidity and vitamin C.
✓ Honey or maple syrup: Provides sweetness without using refined sugar.
✓ Cinnamon has antioxidant and anti-inflammatory effects.
✓ Almonds are high in calcium, magnesium, and vitamin E, which promote bone density and strength.

Benefit for Osteoporosis: Baked apples with cinnamon and almonds are a nutritious and pleasant dessert that promotes bone health. Apples provide dietary fiber, vitamin C, and other antioxidants that improve bone density and strength. Cinnamon includes chemicals that may reduce inflammation and prevent bone loss. Almonds contain calcium, magnesium, and vitamin E, all of which are vital minerals for bone health.

Frozen Banana Pops with Dark Chocolate and Nuts

Ingredients:

- 2 ripe bananas
- 1/4 cup dark chocolate chips
- 2 tablespoons chopped nuts (almonds, walnuts, pistachios)

Instructions:

1. Peel the bananas and then cut them in half crosswise.
2. Insert a popsicle stick into each banana half and set on a baking sheet lined with parchment paper.
3. Melt the dark chocolate chips in a microwave-safe bowl at 30-second intervals, stirring in between, until smooth.
4. Dip each banana half in the melted chocolate, coating evenly.
5. Sprinkle chopped nuts on the chocolate-coated bananas.
6. Place the baking sheet in the freezer for at least 2 hours, or until the chocolate is solid.
7. Serve frozen banana pops as a delightful and healthful dessert.

Nutritional value:

✓ Bananas provide potassium, vitamin B6, and dietary fiber, which are essential for bone health and muscle function.
✓ Dark chocolate contains flavonoids and antioxidants, which may increase bone density and reduce inflammation.
✓ Nuts are high in calcium, magnesium, and healthy fats, which promote bone density and strength.

Benefits for Osteoporosis: These frozen banana pops with dark chocolate and nuts are a tasty and bone-friendly treat. Bananas include potassium, which promotes bone health and controls calcium levels. Dark chocolate contains flavonoids, which may help increase bone density and lower the risk of osteoporosis. Nuts provide calcium, magnesium, and healthy fats that promote bone health and overall well-being.

Yogurt Berry Popsicles

Ingredients:

- 1 cup Greek yogurt
- 1/2 cup mixed berries (strawberries, blueberries, raspberries)
- 1 tablespoon honey or maple syrup
- Popsicle molds

Instructions:

1. In a bowl, stir Greek yogurt and honey or maple syrup until fully incorporated.
2. Gently fold in the mixed berries.
3. Pour the yogurt-berry mixture into popsicle molds, filling them to the top.
4. Place popsicle sticks inside each mold.
5. Place the molds in the freezer for at least 4 hours, or until the popsicles are solid.
6. Once frozen, take the popsicles out of the molds and serve immediately.

Nutritional value:

- ✓ Greek yogurt is high in protein and calcium, which are needed for bone health.
- ✓ Mixed berries are high in antioxidants and vitamin C, which promote collagen formation and bone health.
- ✓ Honey or maple syrup: Provides sweetness without using refined sugar.

Benefits for Osteoporosis: These yogurt berry popsicles are a delicious and bone-friendly dessert. Greek yogurt contains protein and calcium, which are essential for maintaining bone density and strength. Mixed berries provide antioxidants that prevent bone loss and promote general bone health. These popsicles are a healthier option for anyone who are concerned about their bone health because they include no refined sugar.

Almond Date Energy Balls

Ingredients:

- 1 cup almonds
- 1 cup pitted dates
- 1 tablespoon cocoa powder
- 1 tablespoon chia seeds
- 1/2 teaspoon vanilla extract
- Pinch of salt

- Desiccated coconut (for coating, optional)

Instructions:

1. In a food processor, pulse almonds until finely ground.
2. Add pitted dates, cocoa powder, chia seeds, vanilla essence, and salt to a food processor.
3. Process until the ingredients come together into a sticky dough.
4. Roll the dough into little balls with your hands.
5. Optionally, cover the energy balls with desiccated coconut.
6. Place the energy balls on a baking sheet lined with parchment paper and refrigerate for at least 30 minutes to set.
7. Serve chilled for a healthy and energizing dessert.

Nutritional value:

- ✓ Almonds: Calcium, magnesium, and healthy fats are all essential to bone health.
- ✓ Dates are high in potassium, fiber, and antioxidants, which promote bone density and overall health.
- ✓ Cocoa powder contains flavonoids and antioxidants, which may increase bone density and reduce inflammation.
- ✓ Chia seeds include calcium, magnesium, and omega-3 fatty acids, all of which are beneficial to bone health.
- ✓ Desiccated coconut: Enhances flavor and texture.

Benefits for Osteoporosis: These almond date energy balls are a nutritious and enjoyable treat that promotes bone health.

Almonds include calcium and magnesium, two nutrients required for bone density and strength. Dates include potassium and antioxidants that promote bone health and lower the incidence of osteoporosis. Cocoa powder and chia seeds provide additional nutrients and antioxidants that improve bone health.

Baked Pears with Cinnamon and Walnuts

Ingredients:

- 2 ripe pears, halved and cored
- 2 tablespoons chopped walnuts
- 1 tablespoon honey or maple syrup
- 1/2 teaspoon ground cinnamon
- Greek yogurt or vanilla ice cream (for serving, optional)

Instructions:

1. Preheat the oven to 375° Fahrenheit (190° Celsius).

2. Place the pear halves cut side up on a baking sheet lined with parchment paper.
3. In a small bowl, combine the chopped walnuts, honey or maple syrup, and ground cinnamon.
4. Spread the walnut mixture in the center of each pear half.
5. Bake in a preheated oven for 20-25 minutes, or until the pears are soft and the topping is golden brown.
6. Serve the baked pears warm, topped with a dollop of Greek yogurt or a scoop of vanilla ice cream.

Nutritional value:

✓ Pears provide dietary fiber, vitamin C, and antioxidants, which are beneficial to bone health and overall well-being.
✓ Walnuts are high in omega-3 fatty acids, protein, and minerals such as calcium and magnesium, which are beneficial to bone health.
✓ Honey or maple syrup: Provides sweetness without using refined sugar.
✓ Cinnamon has antioxidant and anti-inflammatory effects.

Benefits for Osteoporosis: These baked pears with cinnamon and walnuts make a delicious and bone-friendly dessert. Pears provide dietary fiber, vitamin C, and antioxidants, which promote bone health and digestion. Walnuts include omega-3 fatty acids and minerals such as calcium and magnesium, which are necessary for bone density and strength. This dessert is a healthier option for those concerned about their bone health because it contains no refined sugar.

Spinach Banana Smoothie Bowl

Ingredients:

- 1 ripe banana, frozen
- 1 cup fresh spinach leaves
- 1/2 cup unsweetened almond milk (or any milk of choice)
- 1 tablespoon almond butter
- 1 tablespoon chia seeds
- 1 tablespoon honey or maple syrup (optional)
- Toppings: Sliced bananas, berries, chopped nuts, granola, shredded coconut

Instructions:

1. In a blender, add the frozen banana, spinach leaves, almond milk, almond butter, chia seeds, and honey/maple syrup.
2. Blend until smooth and creamy, adding more almond milk as needed to achieve the desired consistency.
3. Pour the smoothie into a bowl. Garnish with sliced bananas,

berries, chopped almonds, granola, and shredded coconut.

Nutritional value:

- ✓ Banana contains potassium, vitamin B6, and fiber, which are good for bone health and digestion.
- ✓ Spinach: High in calcium, magnesium, and vitamin K, which are necessary for bone density and strength.
- ✓ Almond milk contains calcium and vitamin D, which are essential for preserving bone mass.
- ✓ Almond butter contains healthy fats, protein, and minerals such as calcium and magnesium.
- ✓ Chia seeds are high in calcium, omega-3 fatty acids, and fiber, which promote bone health and digestion.
- ✓ Honey or maple syrup: Provides sweetness without using refined sugar.

Benefits for Osteoporosis: This spinach banana smoothie bowl is a nutritious and delicious dessert that promotes bone health. Bananas include potassium, which promotes bone health and controls calcium levels. Spinach contains calcium, magnesium, and vitamin K, which are necessary elements for bone density and strength. Almond milk and almond butter provide calcium, magnesium, and healthy lipids that promote bone health. Chia seeds include calcium, omega-3 fatty acids, and fiber, which promote general bone health and well-being.

Quinoa Coconut Pudding

Ingredients:

- 1/2 cup uncooked quinoa
- 1 can (13.5 oz) coconut milk
- 2 tablespoons honey or maple syrup
- 1 teaspoon vanilla extract
- Pinch of salt
- Fresh berries for topping (optional)
- Shredded coconut for garnish (optional)

Instructions:

1. Rinse the quinoa with cool water.
2. In a saucepan, mix the quinoa, coconut milk, honey or maple syrup, vanilla extract, and a bit of salt.
3. Bring the mixture to a boil, then reduce to low heat and simmer for 15-20 minutes, or until the quinoa is tender and the mixture thickens.
4. Remove from heat and allow cooling for a few minutes.

5. Serve the quinoa coconut pudding warm or cold garnished with fresh berries and shredded coconut as preferred.

Nutritional value:

- ✓ Quinoa contains protein, fiber, and minerals such as calcium, magnesium, and phosphorus, which are beneficial to bone health.
- ✓ Coconut milk: Provides healthful fats and a creamy texture, which improves the flavor of the pudding.
- ✓ Honey or maple syrup: Provides sweetness without using refined sugar.
- ✓ Vanilla extract enhances flavor without adding calories.
- ✓ Fresh berries and shredded coconut provide additional flavor and texture.

Benefits for Osteoporosis: This quinoa coconut pudding is a nutritious and tasty treat that promotes bone health. Quinoa is a complete protein source with minerals like calcium and magnesium, which are necessary for bone density and strength. Coconut milk contains healthy fats and has a creamy texture, which improves the taste of the pudding. This dessert is a healthier option for those concerned about their bone health because it contains no refined sugar.

Pumpkin Pie Chia Pudding

Ingredients:

- 1/4 cup chia seeds
- 1 cup unsweetened almond milk (or any milk of choice)
- 1/2 cup pumpkin puree
- 2 tablespoons maple syrup or honey
- 1 teaspoon pumpkin pie spice
- 1/2 teaspoon vanilla extract
- Whipped cream or coconut cream for topping (optional)
- Ground cinnamon for garnish (optional)

Instructions:

1. In a mixing bowl, blend chia seeds, almond milk, pumpkin puree, maple syrup or honey, pumpkin pie spice, and vanilla extract until well incorporated.
2. Cover the bowl and refrigerate for at least 2 hours, or overnight, until the chia pudding has thickened.
3. Stir the chia pudding before serving to ensure it has a consistent consistency.
4. Divide the pudding between serving glasses or bowls.
5. Top with whipped cream or coconut cream and, if preferred, crushed cinnamon.

Nutritional value:

- ✓ Chia seeds are high in calcium, omega-3 fatty acids, and fiber, which is good for your bones and digestion.

- ✓ Almond milk contains calcium and vitamin D, which are essential for bone health.
- ✓ Pumpkin puree contains vitamins A, C, and potassium, which promote bone health and overall well-being.
- ✓ Maple syrup or honey: Provides sweetness without using refined sugar.
- ✓ Pumpkin pie spice offers warm, aromatic tastes reminiscent of autumn.

Benefits for Osteoporosis: This pumpkin pie chia pudding is a creamy and tasty treat that helps with bone health. Chia seeds contain calcium, omega-3 fatty acids, and fiber, which are all critical elements for bone density and digestion. Almond milk contains calcium and vitamin D, which are essential for bone health. Pumpkin puree provides vitamins A, C, and potassium, all of which promote bone health and overall well-being.

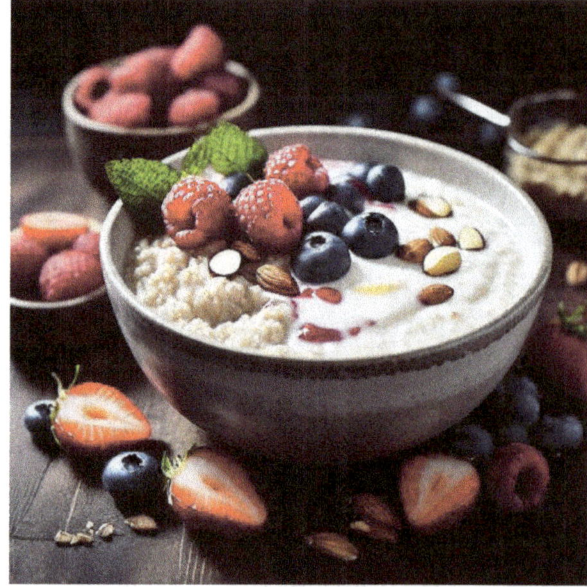

7 DAYS MEAL PLAN

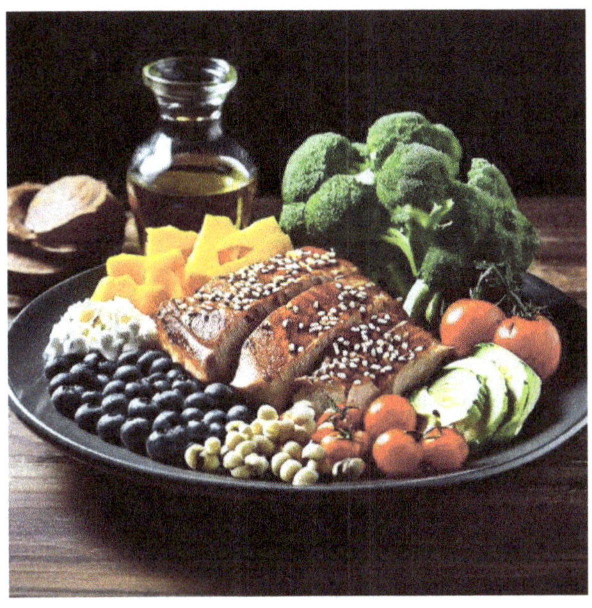

Day 1:

Breakfast: Spinach and Feta Omelette with Whole Wheat Toast

Spinach provides calcium and vitamin K.

Feta cheese offers calcium and protein.

Whole wheat toast provides fiber and magnesium.

Lunch: Quinoa Salad with Grilled Chicken and Avocado

Quinoa is rich in protein and magnesium.

Grilled chicken offers protein and phosphorus.

Avocado provides healthy fats and vitamin K.

Dinner: Baked Salmon with Steamed Broccoli and Brown Rice

Salmon is a source of vitamin D and omega-3 fatty acids.

Broccoli offers calcium and vitamin K.

Brown rice provides fiber and magnesium.

Snack: Greek Yogurt with Mixed Berries

Greek yogurt offers calcium and protein.

Mixed berries provide antioxidants and vitamin C.

Day 2:

Breakfast: Overnight Oats with Almond Milk, Chia Seeds, and Sliced Banana

Overnight oats provide fiber and magnesium.

Almond milk offers calcium and vitamin D.

Chia seeds provide omega-3 fatty acids and phosphorus.

Lunch: Turkey and Avocado Wrap with Whole Grain Tortilla

Turkey offers protein and phosphorus.

Avocado provides healthy fats and vitamin K.

Whole grain tortilla offers fiber and magnesium.

Dinner: Lentil Soup with Kale and Whole Grain Bread

Lentils are rich in protein and magnesium.

Kale provides calcium and vitamin K.

Whole grain bread offers fiber and phosphorus.

Snack: Carrot Sticks with Hummus

Carrots provide vitamin A and calcium.

Hummus offers protein and magnesium.

Day 3:

Breakfast: Greek Yogurt Parfait with Granola and Mixed Berries

Greek yogurt offers calcium and protein.

Granola provides fiber and magnesium.

Mixed berries offer antioxidants and vitamin C.

Lunch: Spinach Salad with Grilled Shrimp, Strawberries, and Walnuts

Spinach provides calcium and vitamin K.

Grilled shrimp offers protein and phosphorus.

Strawberries provide antioxidants and vitamin C.

Walnuts offer omega-3 fatty acids and magnesium.

Dinner: Chicken Stir-Fry with Broccoli, Bell Peppers, and Brown Rice

Chicken offers protein and phosphorus.

Broccoli provides calcium and vitamin K.

Bell peppers offer vitamin C.

Brown rice provides fiber and magnesium.

Snack: Cottage Cheese with Pineapple Chunks

Cottage cheese offers calcium and protein.

Pineapple provides vitamin C and manganese.

Day 4:

Breakfast: Whole Grain Pancakes with Greek Yogurt and Blueberries

Whole grain pancakes provide fiber and magnesium.

Greek yogurt offers calcium and protein.

Blueberries provide antioxidants and vitamin C.

 Quinoa Stuffed Bell Peppers with Ground Turkey and Spinach

Quinoa provides protein and magnesium.

Ground turkey offers protein and phosphorus.

Spinach provides calcium and vitamin K.

Bell peppers offer vitamin C.

Dinner: Baked Cod with Asparagus and Quinoa Pilaf

Cod provides protein and vitamin D.

Asparagus offers calcium and vitamin K.

Quinoa pilaf provides protein and magnesium.

Snack: Sliced Apple with Almond Butter

Apple offers fiber and vitamin C.

Almond butter provides protein and calcium.

Day 5:

Breakfast: Scrambled Tofu with Spinach and Whole Wheat Toast

Tofu offers protein and calcium.

Spinach provides calcium and vitamin K.

Whole wheat toast provides fiber and magnesium.

Lunch: Lentil and Vegetable Soup with Whole Grain Crackers

Lentils provide protein and magnesium.

Mixed vegetables offer calcium and vitamin K.

Whole grain crackers provide fiber and phosphorus.

Dinner: Grilled Steak with Sweet Potato Mash and Green Beans

Steak offers protein and phosphorus.

Sweet potatoes provide vitamin A and potassium.

Green beans offer calcium and vitamin K.

Snack: Greek Yogurt Smoothie with Mango and Spinach

Greek yogurt offers calcium and protein.

Mango provides vitamin C.

Spinach offers calcium and vitamin K.

Day 6:

Breakfast: Whole Grain Waffles with Yogurt and Sliced Strawberries

Whole grain waffles provide fiber and magnesium.

Yogurt offers calcium and protein.

Strawberries provide antioxidants and vitamin C.

Chickpeas provide protein and magnesium.

Feta cheese offers calcium and protein.

Cucumber and tomatoes provide vitamin C.

Dinner: Baked Chicken Breast with Roasted Brussels sprouts and Quinoa

Chicken breast offers protein and phosphorus.

Brussels sprouts provide calcium and vitamin K.

Quinoa offers protein and magnesium.

Snack: Celery Sticks with Peanut Butter

Celery provides calcium and vitamin K.

Peanut butter offers protein and magnesium.

Day 7:

Breakfast: Banana Almond Butter Smoothie with Spinach and Flaxseeds

Banana offers potassium and fiber.

Almond butter provides protein and calcium.

Spinach offers calcium and vitamin K.

Flaxseeds provide omega-3 fatty acids and magnesium.

Lunch: Turkey and Swiss Cheese Sandwich on Whole Grain Bread

Turkey offers protein and phosphorus.

Swiss cheese provides calcium and protein.

Whole grain bread offers fiber and magnesium.

Dinner: Salmon Salad with Mixed Greens, Avocado, and Balsamic Vinaigrette

Salmon provides protein and vitamin D.

Mixed greens offer calcium and vitamin K.

Avocado provides healthy fats and potassium.

Snack: Greek Yogurt with Honey and Almonds

Greek yogurt offers calcium and protein.

Honey provides natural sweetness.

Almonds offer protein and magnesium.

This 7-day meal plan provides a variety of nutrient-rich foods to support bone health, including calcium-rich foods, vitamin D sources, protein, magnesium and phosphorus, vitamin K, and antioxidant-rich foods. Remember to consult with a healthcare professional or dietitian before making significant changes to your diet, especially if you have specific health concerns or dietary restrictions.

Dear Readers,

As an author passionate about promoting health and well-being among seniors, I am thrilled to share my latest creation with you - the "Osteoporosis Diet Cookbook for Seniors." Crafting this cookbook has been a labor of love, and my ultimate goal is to empower you with delicious and nutritious recipes tailored to support your bone health journey.

Your feedback is incredibly valuable to me. As you explore the recipes and delve into the wealth of information provided, I kindly ask for your honest reviews on Amazon. Your reviews not only help me understand how the cookbook has resonated with you but also assist other seniors in making informed decisions about their health.

Whether you found a particular recipe especially delightful, discovered a helpful tip, or simply enjoyed the overall experience of using the cookbook, your thoughts matter. Your reviews not only motivate me to continue creating content that serves your needs but also contribute to building a supportive community dedicated to embracing a healthy lifestyle.

Thank you for considering sharing your thoughts with me and fellow readers. Your feedback fuels my passion for spreading knowledge and inspiration for healthier living among seniors.

Warm regards,

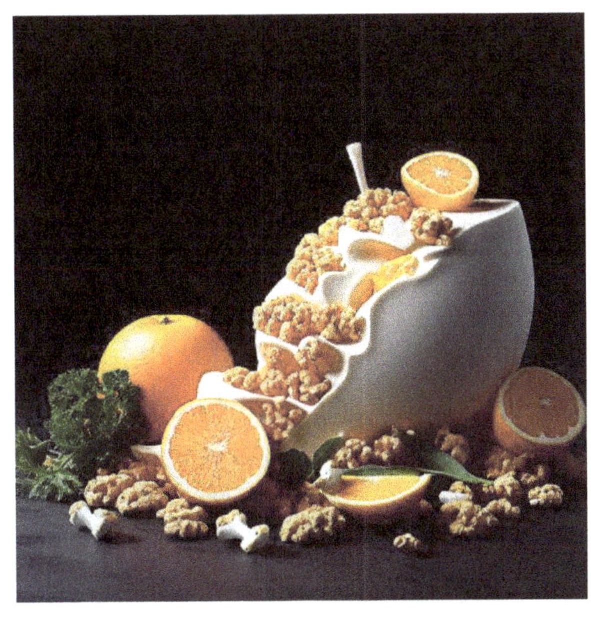

CONCLUSION

Finally, the Osteoporosis Diet Cookbook for Seniors provides complete and practical guidance for maintaining bone health through nutrition. This cookbook, which emphasizes calcium-rich foods, vitamin D sources, protein, magnesium, phosphorus, vitamin K, and antioxidant-rich foods, offers a variety of delicious and healthy recipes designed specifically for seniors treating osteoporosis.

Throughout this cookbook, we've looked at a variety of breakfasts, lunches, dinners, snacks, desserts, juices, and smoothies that not only fuel the body but also aid in strengthening bones and lowering the chance of fracture. From substantial oatmeal bowls to tasty salads, warm soups, and delectable desserts, each recipe is meticulously designed to supply the necessary nutrients for bone health.

By including these recipes in your regular food plan, you may make proactive efforts to increase bone density, preserve bone strength, and enhance overall health. Whether you want to avoid osteoporosis or manage its symptoms, eating nutrient-dense meals is essential for supporting bone health and lowering the risk of fractures.

Remember that, in addition to a balanced diet, regular exercise, enough sunlight exposure, and avoiding smoking and excessive alcohol use are all important for maintaining strong and healthy bones. By combining these lifestyle variables with the dishes and suggestions in this cookbook, you can regain control of your bone health and live a full and active life long into your senior years.

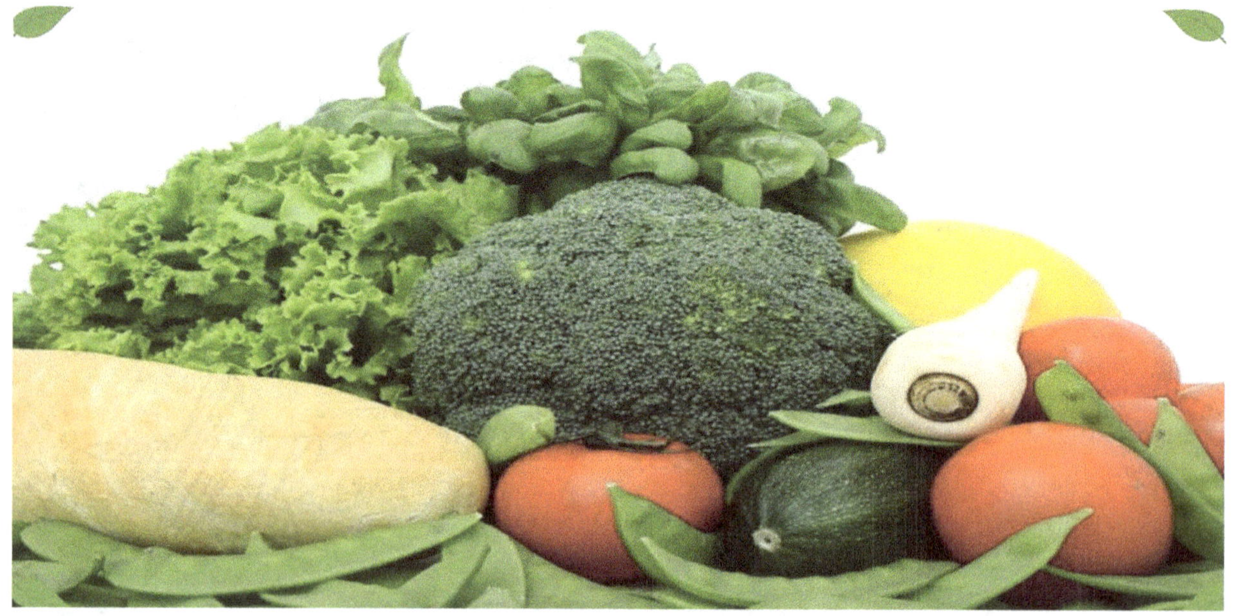